HEALTH IN

Lori Reid is a professional hand analyst consulted by people from all over the world. She is regularly featured as an expert in her field on both national radio and television, having contributed to such programmes as BBC1's *Bodymatters* and ITV's *The Time . . . The Place*, but is perhaps best known in the South-West for her many TV and radio broadcasts such as the popular celebrity series *Zodiac & Co.* Lori Reid has written articles for several national and international journals and newspapers, and is a regular contributor of features for women's magazines. She has written a number of books on hand analysis and other related subjects.

By the same author

HEALTH IN YOUR HANDS

Lori Reid

Aquarian/Thorsons
An Imprint of HarperCollinsPublishers

The Aquarian Press
An Imprint of HarperCollins*Publishers*
77-85 Fulham Palace Road,
Hammersmith, London W6 8JB

Published by The Aquarian Press 1993
1 3 5 7 9 10 8 6 4 2

A catalogue record for this book
is available from the British Library

ISBN 1 85538 182 6

Printed in Great Britain by
HarperCollinsManufacturing Glasgow

To my best friend
Pauline Champness
best counsellor
best clinical psychologist
best healer of troubled minds

CONTENTS

AUTHOR'S NOTE

Supplements, remedies and massage techniques outlined in this book are suggested as a reference source, not as a medical guide. Herbs contain active properties, some of which have a powerful effect even if taken in minute doses. Similarly, under certain circumstances, massaging may be counter-productive. If you wish to follow the therapies, if you are suffering with a medical condition or are on prescribed medication, you are recommended to consult your doctor for advice before you begin.

Of the vitamins and minerals mentioned, the daily recommended international units should not be exceeded even by those enjoying good health. The tissue salts, often given in abbreviation throughout the book, form part of the twelve minerals that make up the biochemic remedies according to Dr. Schuessler's system. The twelve are as follows:

1. Calc. Fluor.	. . .	Calcium Fluoride
2. Calc. Phos.	. . .	Calcium Phosphate
3. Calc. Sulph.	. . .	Calcium Sulphate
4. Ferr. Phos.	. . .	Phosphate of Iron
5. Kali. Mur.	. . .	Potassium Chloride
6. Kali. Phos.	. . .	Potassium Phosphate
7. Kali. Sulph.	. . .	Potassium Sulphate
8. Mag. Phos.	. . .	Magnesium Phosphate
9. Nat. Mur.	. . .	Sodium Chloride
10. Nat. Phos.	. . .	Sodium Phosphate
11. Nat. Sulph.	. . .	Sodium Sulphate
12. Silica	. . .	Silicic Oxide

INTRODUCTION

There is little doubt that a connection exists between our hands and our health. As a matter of course, doctors routinely consult the hands of their patients not only for taking the pulse at the wrist, but also for a variety of symptoms that will back up their diagnosis of disease.

For example, listless hands will often accompany a lack of energy or a loss of motivation. Tremor is linked with hormonal problems, with toxicity and with diseases of the nervous system. Discolouration and abnormal temperature may be caused by faulty oxygenation, by problems of the cardio-vascular system, by feverishness, by shock, by an imbalance of the endocrine system, and a whole host of other conditions which are recognized as producing corresponding symptoms in the hand. Centuries of studying and analysing hands have shown emphatically that these links exist, that signs and symptoms of our inherent predisposition to disease as well as the possibility of future ill-health imprint their subtle clues all over our fingers and palms.

We now know that it is because our palms contain a vast concentration of nerve endings, more so than any other part of our anatomy (with the exception of the soles of our feet), that they make such superb registers upon which our nervous responses and biochemical messages may be imprinted. Moreover, in recent times scientific research on the hand has established a relationship between unusual fingerprints or skin markings and genetic or congenital abnormalities. This link is now widely recognized and may well be of great value in genetic counselling as well as an aid to general medical diagnosis.

When understood, all of these messages, these various features and formations in our palms and fingers, can give valuable clues about the state of our health. These markings highlight our resistance, our vitality; show tell-tale hints of the build-up of toxins, reveal imbalances and wear-and-tear; give warnings of potential danger spots; and generally present a picture of our constitutional weak links, our predisposition to disease.

Health in your Hands, then, traces and explains the meaning of the markings that relate to your health and well-being. It shows how your basic personality type, revealed by the shape of your hand, influences your ideas, your attitudes, your way of life and consequently your state of health. It first takes a broad look at the physical characteristics of your nails, of your fingerprints, of the colour and temperature of your hands, and then a microscopic view of the finer lines and formations that make up the markings in your palms. And at each stage not only will these markings be interpreted but, wherever possible, relevant advice will be given on preventive measures together with invaluable information on nutrition and diet. And because this book is fundamentally about preventing disease by picking up early clues about your health in your hand, the chapters on reflexology and massage are designed not only as another form of early detection, but also to promote good health and well-being on a daily basis.

But throughout it must be borne in mind that you must never make the mistake of diagnosing from the hand alone. However, knowing how to interpret the signs and markings in your hands means that you can become aware of the subtle changes that are taking place in your body. And because many of these lines and markings are in constant flux, appearing and disappearing according to your circumstances, understanding the particular configurations will allow you to monitor and intervene in your own health. You can, in effect, allow your habits and lifestyle to render you vulnerable to illness, or you can choose to maintain your good health and actively prevent the development of disease. In this way, you can literally take your health into your own hands.

I

The Four Psychological Types

We all know that our characters and personalities contribute a good deal to the pattern of our health and well-being in life. The way we each cope with the stresses and strains of modern living depends to a great extent on our attitudes, our hopes and aspirations. Our lifestyles, too, equally responsible for our susceptibility to disease, are likewise dependent on our characters. Hence, the bottom line when it comes to assessing aspects of health must lie in our own psychological make-up.

Just as our genes determine the colour of our eyes or whether we will have straight or curly hair, so our chromosomal blueprint will lay down the shape of our hands, the patterns that we recognize as fingerprints and the major lines that are found criss-crossing the palm. And just as genetically we might be classified as blond, brunette or redhead which, some would argue, would reflect a great deal about our personalities, so, too, to the trained hand analyst our hands can be classified into one of four types each of which will give a good deal of information about ourselves and about what makes us tick.

Fundamentally, our hands may be described as living registers which record all manner of data about ourselves: how we think and behave, how we work and love, relate and interact with others, our hopes and dreams, our ambitions and aspirations, our conscious and subconscious motivations, our preferences, innate gifts and talents, inclinations, tendencies and predispositions, our actions and reactions, what we've done in the past and, consequently, what we are likely to do in the future.

Grouping all hands into merely four types may seem oversimplistic but this does at least allow us to make certain preliminary generalizations about people. More importantly, rather like the chicken-wire structure upon which a sculptor starts to form his model, each category of hands provides a solid framework upon which we can *begin* to build a profile of those belonging to each group, together with their attitudes to health and tendency to disease. Once the general type has been established we then have a route in to analysing the specific in terms of skin markings and line formations.

These four hand categories, named after the elements of **Earth, Air, Fire** and **Water** are, of necessity, 'pure' types and few hands will be expected to correspond to them exactly in every detail. After all, each single hand is uniquely individual – there are no two alike, not even our right hands match our left ones perfectly. Nevertheless, uniqueness apart, your hands should more or less conform to one or other of the four types, and if not exactly, then enough at least to classify them so that your *basic* temperament and fundamental nature can be charted. If, however, your hand shape seems to fall between two categories, it simply means that you possess a combination of the qualities represented by both types.

THE EARTH HAND

APPEARANCE
Characteristically, the Earth hand is made up of a squarish palm topped by short, blunt-tipped fingers (see Figure 1). There are likely to be few lines in the palm – only three or four in many cases – but these will be strong, thus giving the hand an uncluttered look and a general feeling of positive strength. Arched or looped fingerprints invariably go with this type.

TEMPERAMENT AND WAY OF LIFE
Earth-handed people are traditional at heart: solid, stable, down-to-earth characters. Practical, hard-working and level-headed, they like a routine, orderly life. Definitely outdoor types, they hate being cooped up inside for long. More rural than urban, they are close

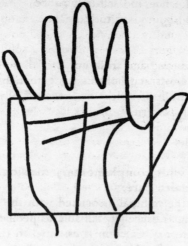

Fig. 1
THE EARTH HAND

to the land and have an affinity with Nature and, in particular, enjoy a special rapport with plants and animals.

Common sense, practicality and a rational tried-and-tested approach to life sums up the temperament of Earth-handed folk. Dogged in their persistence and perseverance, they have no time for flighty, fanciful theories or unrealistic schemes. Physical activity characterizes those belonging to the Earth-handed category.

Earth type susceptibilities:
- worry
- bowel or intestinal problems
- skin ailments
- problems with joints
- physical fatigue

Avoid:
- stress produced by erratic routines
- nervous tension
- weight gain

- physical indolence and self-indulgence
- negative feelings and attitudes

Encourage:
- plenty of exercise and fresh air
- outdoor interests and hobbies e.g. gardening, walking
- regularity within lifestyle
- a good sleep pattern
- a positive attitude
- a healthy diet

Associations with complementary medicine and alternative health care:
- Calcium is the mineral associated with the Earth hand shape and, as such, is especially suitable to people whose hands fall into this category. Calcium is essential to the production and maintainance of teeth and bones. It assists in blood clotting, promotes the healthy action of the heart and helps to maintain good muscle tone. A deficiency causes tooth decay and softening of the bones as in the condition osteoporosis. In certain cases irritability, depression and insomnia (hence the advice to take a hot, milky drink before bedtime) can also result from an imbalance of calcium. Excess calcium can lead to stiffness of the joints, kidney stones and in extreme conditions, to cardio-vascular problems including arteriosclerosis, or hardening of the arteries.
- Amongst the tissue salts, the calcium family includes calcium fluoride, calcium phosphate and calcium sulphate. Other mineral supplements include calcium ascorbate which combines Vitamin C for easy absorption into the system, calcium aspartate and calcium gluconate.
- Kelp is one of the richest sources of calcium; so, too, are cheese and other dairy products as well as almonds. Fish such as sardines and whitebait, where the bones are also eaten, provide a good supply of the mineral, too.
- Magnesium and Vitamin D assist the absorption and deployment of calcium in the body.
- Violet, rose, grapes, willow and comfrey are all associated with the Earth category.

THE AIR HAND

APPEARANCE

The Air hand is recognized by its square palm and long fingers (see Figure 2). The palm itself will contain several lines – at least a good few more than the bare essentials – and these will be characteristically clear and well-defined. Looped fingerprints will be the predominant pattern here. All in all, with its clearly formed, well-constructed but not necessarily overly heavy lines, the Air hand has about it a certain 'wiry' look.

TEMPERAMENT AND WAY OF LIFE

Forever turning things over to see how they work, Air-handed people have lively, inquisitive minds that make them eternal students, always wanting to know, to investigate, to learn and find out. Their mercurial mentality thrives on communications and in life, as well as at work, they need variety and, more importantly, they need 'Buzz'.

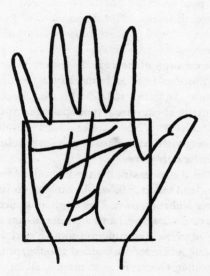

Fig. 2
THE AIR HAND

Characteristically, people who possess the Air hand are notoriously curious about their world and about what makes things work. Chatty and friendly, their minds are constantly ticking over and, because they are quick learners, they have a short attention span and a low boredom threshold. Consequently, Air-handed folk need plenty of interests to keep them stimulated and amused throughout their lives. Mental activity is the key to the Air category.

Air type susceptibilities:
- headaches
- a delicate nervous system
- respiratory problems
- ear, nose and throat complaints
- colds and chills
- mental fatigue

Avoid:
- being stuck in a rut
- too many irons in the fire
- nervous tension
- mental exhaustion

Encourage:
- healthy exchange of news and views
- flexible routines both at home and at work
- the pursuit of intellectual activities e.g. reading, writing
- regular physical exercise – perhaps team games, aerobics, gym

Associations with complementary medicine and alternative health care:
- Because of the incessant demands on their mental and nervous systems, Air-handed folk would do well to turn to magnesium when they feel run-down. This mineral is particularly beneficial to owners of the Air hand because it assists in the smooth running of nerve cell function and so acts as a nerve soother and muscle relaxant. Air-handed people are notorious for their nervous energy and fidgety minds, all of which upsets the delicate balance of this mineral and depletes whatever reserves they have of it in their bodies. Stress and nervous activity are

prime expenders of magnesium, with the resulting deficit producing a chicken-and-egg situation: nervous activity = drain on magnesium = jangly nerves = nervous activity. A deficiency of magnesium can lead to over-excitability, nervous tension, headaches, neuralgic shooting pains, muscular twitches, cramps and all manner of nervous disorders and instability.

- Amongst the tissue salts magnesium phosphate is the nerve restorative. Other mineral supplements include magnesium ascorbate which combines with Vitamin C for easy absorption, magnesium aspartate and magnesium gluconate.
- Kelp is a particularly good source of magnesium but other foods rich in the mineral include nuts and grains, especially almonds, peanuts, brazils, wheatbran and brown rice.
- Lavender, marjoram, mint, ash and elderflower are associated with the Air category.

THE FIRE HAND

APPEARANCE

Like the Earth hand, the Fire hand, too, has short fingers but its most distinguishing characteristic is its longer palm (see Figure 3). This hand contains strong lines of which there are a goodly amount. Whorled fingerprints are also associated with this category.

TEMPERAMENT AND WAY OF LIFE

Physically active and dynamic, these people are always on the go. They need adventure and excitement in their lives as fuel for their super-abundance of energy and drive – which they often channel into sports. The life and soul of the party, they are wonderful with people, spreading enthusiasm and inspiration wherever they go. These high-profile types often become performers and entertainers, drawn like moths to the glare of the spotlight.

Fire types like to be right at the centre of the action. Happiest when living life in the fast lane, they do have a tendency to burn the candle at both ends and to push themselves to the very limits of their mental and physical capacities.

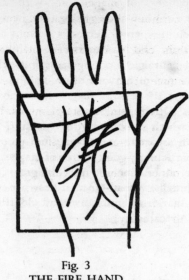

Fig. 3
THE FIRE HAND

Fire type susceptibilities:
- accidents and injuries from burns and sharp objects
- cardio-vascular problems
- backache and problems of the spinal column
- chills and feverishness
- mental and physical burnout

Avoid:
- mental or physical overload by over-enthusiastically taking on too much
- food that is overly rich or spicy
- too much alcohol or other stimulants
- sudden, dramatic moods
- excessive haste and careless, precipitate action that can lead to accidents and injury
- leaving things to the last minute
- restlessness
- putting on weight

Encourage:

- peace and harmony through e.g. yoga, meditation, breathing techniques
- regular sports and workouts into which energies can be channelled
- the maintenance of an even pace at home and at work

Associations with complementary medicine and alternative health care:

- Potassium is the mineral that comes to mind when considering the dynamic Fire category. It is particularly associated with the Fire types because these are physically active people, little whirlwinds that are always on the go, and potassium is a mineral which works directly on the action of the muscles, helping to keep them toned and promoting their efficient functioning. But as well as being physical, Fire-handed folk use a lot of mental energy, too, and it is here that potassium's other role, that as a nerve nutrient, comes into play. Thus it is that those belonging to this category can benefit greatly from supplements of this mineral, particularly at those times when demands on their mental and physical reserves are at a premium – during exams, for example, or training for an important race or even rehearsing day and night the lead role in, say, *Hedda Gabler*. One of the first symptoms of a deficiency of potassium is listlessness and general muscular weakness. A dry, rough, scaly skin lacking elasticity, brittle nails, pains in the joints and limbs, woolly-mindedness, depression and irregular action of the heart may all be associated with a deficiency or imbalance of potassium.
- Amongst the tissue salts, the potassium family includes potassium chloride, potassium phosphate and potassium sulphate. Other mineral supplements that may prove especially beneficial are potassium gluconate and potassium aspartate.
- Fish and seaweed, in the form of kelp, are rich sources of potassium. Fruit and vegetables such as bananas, raisins, dates, avocados, carrots, cabbage and spinach all contain large concentrations of the mineral.
- Peppermint tea, hops, onions, leeks, rosemary, sage, dandelion and borage are all associated with the Fire category.

THE WATER HAND

APPEARANCE

The Water hand is unmistakable in its appearance principally because of its long, often lean and graceful look (see Figure 4). An oblong palm topped by long tapering fingers is characteristic of this type. Invariably, the palm is covered by many fine lines giving the appearance of a cobweb effect. Loop fingerprint patterns are, as a rule, found on the fingertips of the Water hand.

TEMPERAMENT AND WAY OF LIFE

Water-handed people are the most sensitive and gentle of the four types. Poetic and romantic, they are artistic and musically gifted.

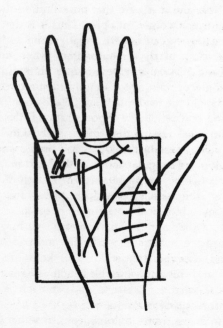

Fig. 4
THE WATER HAND

They are cultured and refined, have good taste but tend to be rather unworldly, living a great deal with their heads in the clouds. A beautiful hand tends to reflect an elegant body and indeed many of these people are found in the fashion world, the modelling business and the beauty industry. The world of the arts and music is also heavily populated by Water-handed folk.

Highly-strung and vulnerable to the stresses and strains of modern living, these people function best in a peaceful and harmonious environment. Pressure, or any sort of competitive situation, is actively detrimental to the Water-handed group.

Water type susceptibilities:
- sensitive digestive system
- depression, neuroses, obsessional behaviour and other such psychological conditions
- delicate skin
- allergic reactions
- rheumatic ailments
- delicate immune system
- complications of the reproductive system
- low physical stamina and resources
- addiction

Avoid:
- stress through competition
- mood swings, especially depression, melancholia or morbidity
- repressing emotions
- irrational or over-imaginative fears
- running away or escapism through drugs or alcohol
- negativity

Encourage:
- expression of the feelings
- peace and harmony in both the domestic and working environment
- confidence through the development of one's skills and talents
- a rational approach to problems
- gentle sports e.g. swimming, sailing, ice-skating, dancing
- balance and moderation in all things

Associations with complementary medicine and alternative health care:

- Because of its associations with water, sodium is the mineral that applies to this category. Sodium is responsible for regulating tissue fluids and helps to maintain the water balance in the body. Too little salt in the body is as bad as too much and can lead to muscular cramps, whilst an excess can upset the cardiovascular system, causing high blood pressure and irregular heart rhythm. Today, sodium chloride, in the form of table salt, is all too prevalent in the Western diet, especially in processed and fast foods, so a reduction, rather than a supplement, is perhaps advisable nowadays. Historically, however, the picture was quite different. Because fresh or natural foods contain little sodium, salt was at a premium and held in such high regard that people were often paid for their labour in bags of salt. Sodium is lost naturally through bodily fluids such as tears and sweat and too great a loss will result in dehydration, a serious condition which can lead to severe complications. So important is it to maintain the correct level of this mineral that in hot climates where people are likely to perspire excessively, salt tablets are recommended to restore its balance in the system. Apart from regulating the water balance, sodium also assists in the production of hydrochloric acid which is essential to the digestive process and as such is helpful to Water-handed folk, many of whom have a predisposition to gastric and intestinal upsets. And because it is also an acid neutralizer, it is useful in the prevention of rheumatic conditions, another vulnerable area in the health of those belonging to this category. Furthermore, sodium's role in both glandular activity and in the control of nerve functioning confirms its association with the Water category whose members are particularly prone to headaches, to nausea, to apathy and moodiness accompanied by feelings of despondency and hopelessness, to watery eyes and to allergic conditions such as hay fever. Indeed, many of these symptoms are the very ones which are associated with an imbalance of this mineral.
- Supplements of tissue salts belonging to the sodium family include sodium chloride, sodium phosphate and sodium sulphate.

- These days a deficiency of sodium is rare in our diets but foods containing a particularly high concentration of the mineral include cheeses and green olives.
- Verbena, tarragon, witch hazel, geranium and lime are all associated with the Water category.

THE FEEL OF THE HAND

Apart from the four general types, the actual feel of your hand can give lots of clues about your health. Whether it is rough as leather or smooth as silk, feels hard as rock or soft as butter, all depends on the texture of your skin and the consistency of your hand. As always, however, try not to make assumptions about your health simply by the feel of your hand alone; any clues that you might pick up in this way *must* be corroborated by other evidence found elsewhere, either in the lines, the nails or the skin ridge patterns. Even then, a diagnosis *must not* be attempted by anyone who is medically unqualified.

IDEAL HAND CONSISTENCY
Ideally, the best sort of consistency for a hand is one where the muscular tone is springy and elastic, not too hard nor too soft. Such a hand denotes a good, vibrant, healthy constitution. Resistance to ill-health and an ability to recuperate quickly and easily following any bout of illness is suggested by a resilient hand which responds like rubber to the touch.

HARD HANDS
Hands that are hard as steel belong to emotionally unyielding types. Their owners are hard workers indeed, the sort who don't seem to lose a single day's work in their lives through physical ill-health. In fact, they are the very types who don't appear to be aware of their nervous systems at all. Insensitivity is their downfall and because they find it difficult to express themselves emotionally, they tend to repress their feelings and thus become prone to the kinds of psychological disorders associated with what might be called emotional constipation.

VERY SOFT, DOUGHY HANDS

The converse of the hard hand is the soft, doughy hand, the sort that when it is held feels like a ball of uncooked pastry. This type of hand with its flabby muscular tone denotes a lack of energy and psychologically is considered to belong to an indolent and self-indulgent individual, someone who does not enjoy any sort of physical activity – unless, that is, it leads to some kind of self-gratification. Perhaps the term 'couch potato' might fit this type well. Physiologically, the soft, doughy hand is characteristic of a lack of vitality and is associated with an imbalance of the thyroid gland. And because here the constitution is not robust, owners of these very soft hands tend to be more vulnerable than most to health disorders.

PODGY HANDS

Obesity often leaves its characteristic mark in the hands in the form of very podgy bottom phalanges to the fingers (see Figure 5a). This, too, is another sign of indolence and sensuality. Sensible diet which can control the weight problem will also help to reduce the podginess of the fingers. More difficult to tackle, though, are the little fatty deposits that are found also on the basal phalanges but this time on the *backs* of the fingers (see Figure 5b). These show that the weight problem is a long-standing affair, possibly having started way back in the individual's childhood, and thus will need greater determination if the excess weight is to be shed.

SUPPLE HANDS

Suppleness is as important a measure as consistency. Flexible hands reflect a flexible nature; thus the individual is able to take the vagaries of life in her stride; he or she is likely to be more tolerant and ride the storms, so to speak. Such people tend to be what is popularly known as 'laid back': relaxed, more able to adjust mentally, physically and emotionally to the demands of the situation and, as such, less vulnerable to life-threatening diseases.

STIFF HANDS

Unlike their more supple-handed colleagues, those who possess stiff hands (unless of course stiffened by disease) hold a feeling of

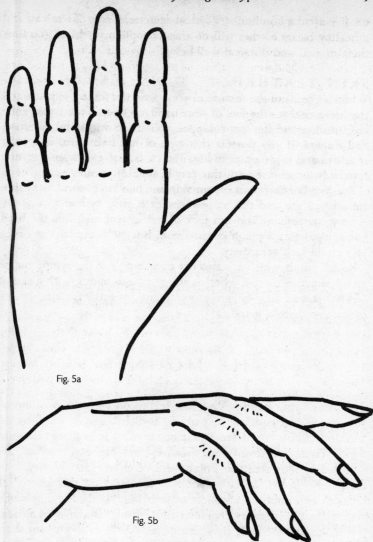

Fig. 5a

Fig. 5b

inner tension and pent-up frustration. People with stiff, hard hands tend to drive themselves too hard; they may be over-ambitious, workaholic perhaps, and thus may well be prone to the stress-related diseases which include hypertension and other serious cardio-vascular conditions. Physical exercise, plenty of fresh air and a healthy balanced diet will do these people a world of good for their mental and physical well-being.

SKIN TEXTURE

When it comes to the texture of your skin, the finer it appears and the more delicate the feel of your hand in general, the weaker the constitution and the less equipped you are to withstand infection and disease. If you possess this type of hand you are, as a rule, sensitive and easily upset in life. Thus it is that a delicate immune system is associated with this fragile type of hand.

The rougher and coarser your skin and hand in general, the more robust you are and the more resistant is your system to disease. A very coarse hand shows a lack of refinement and, like the hard hand, highlights a tough constitution. But be aware that at times you could lack sensitivity.

Rough hands which are also dry can be one of the symptoms of an underactive thyroid whereas shiny smooth hands, with a satiny feel to them, may be symptomatic of hyperthyroidism, or an overactive thyroid gland.

THE MOUNTS

The feel of your hand has a good deal to do with the padding of your palm. Notice how the padding is distributed in the form of 'cushions', little raised areas that occur at various places in your hand. These are known as **mounts** and because mounts are believed to represent the storehouses of energy and vitality, it is their very quality, development and construction that give vital clues to two important aspects of your life. Firstly, they highlight your salient personality characteristics, strengths and weaknesses, if you like, and secondly, they provide tell-tale hints about your state of health and general predisposition to disease.

For easy identification, the mounts have been named after the planets – not just arbitrarily though, for indeed those who know anything about classical mythology would instantly recognize that behind the names lies a wealth of meaning that reflects character

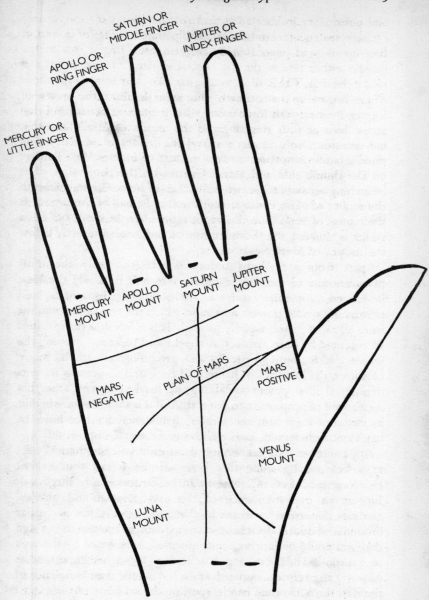

SATURN OR
MIDDLE FINGER

JUPITER OR
INDEX FINGER

APOLLO OR
RING FINGER

MERCURY OR
LITTLE FINGER

MERCURY
MOUNT

APOLLO
MOUNT

SATURN
MOUNT

JUPITER
MOUNT

MARS
NEGATIVE

PLAIN OF MARS

MARS
POSITIVE

VENUS
MOUNT

LUNA
MOUNT

Fig. 6

and personality in shorthand form.

There are eight mounts in all, as illustrated in Figure 6: four at the top of your palm roughly beneath each finger, two in the middle, either side of the flat central expanse of your palm, and two at the base. The four across the top take their names from those of the fingers so that beneath your index is found the mount of Jupiter. Beneath your middle finger lies the mount of Saturn. Lying at the root of your ring finger is the mount of Apollo and that beneath your little finger is called the mount of Mercury. The middle band comprises the two mounts of Mars – Mars Positive on the thumb side and Mars Negative on the percussion edge. Stretching between these two is the Plain of Mars. Directly beneath the mount of Mars Positive, and forming the ball of the thumb, is the mount of Venus. On the opposite side lies the mount of Luna which is situated just above your wrist and located directly below the mount of Mars Negative.

Apart from the Venus mount which is usually the most pronounced and the Saturn mount which is normally the least developed, someone with a well-balanced disposition and personality would possess a hand in which the rest of the mounts were all more or less equally padded. This is because the qualities represented by each area act as checks and balances, keeping the whole system, both physically and psychologically, in harmony. However, the majority of hands will be found to possess mounts of unequal development containing one, maybe even two, areas that appear out of proportion to the rest. And it is these areas, whether by virtue of their dominance or of their deficiency, that hold the key to our characters, personalities and natural disposition.

Any mount in your hand that is **dominant** will automatically act as a beacon, signalling that here will be found your salient characteristics. But any that are **huge or unusually large** will suggest an over-abundance of the psychological and physical qualities that are represented by that area. Equally, if a particular mount is obviously **deficient** in comparison to the rest, it is a sign that you could be lacking those qualities represented by the area in question. Thus, noticing a deficiency is just as important as noticing an over-development, as each will reflect an imbalance in the nature. With some hands, spotting the odd one out is easy: a dominant mount will stand out and overshadow the rest, so that will be the one to concentrate on. And if there are two apparently dominant mounts, the qualities that each represents will be found to be prominently combined in that individual's nature. Other hands may seem to be totally flat, with no single mount standing out at all, and in these cases it will be other factors, such as the shape of the hand, the fingerprints or lines in the palm, for example, that will hold the relevant clues concerning matters of health.

THE MOUNT OF VENUS

Your mount of Venus, or thenar eminence, lies directly below your thumb and forms that part of the palm that is known as the ball of the thumb. It is bounded by a semi-circular line called the Life line. When the mount is large and full, the Life line may sweep well out towards the centre of the palm. But when deficient and meagre in construction, the Life line may skirt round in a tight arc closely hugging the root of the thumb. In most hands this will be found to be the biggest of the mounts and so should not as a rule be interpreted as the dominant area unless it visibly towers above the rest, or appears to cover an inordinately large expanse of palm.

Physical characteristics: Because this area covers the radial artery as it enters the palm from the wrist as well as the muscles controlling movement of the thumb, the amount of padding and the actual quality of this mount will give information regarding your resilience and vitality. Hence, rude health, robustness, ability to bounce back, whether physically or psychologically, and powers of recuperation are all marked here. To test for vitality and good health, press the tip of your thumb into the Venus mount and, on releasing it, notice how the padding responds to the pressure. If the mount readily springs back, your health, vitality and recuperative powers are good. If the mount is flabby and retains the indentation, your health may be under par and your resistance to disease poor. If the mount is so hard that you are unable to dent the surface at all, you are probably someone with a constitution of iron. In addition to the physical characteristics, the extent of your affection and instinctive sexuality are also denoted by the construction and development of this mount. Venusians are characterized by their happy, friendly and optimistic attitudes to life.

Psychological profile: Expect a strong degree of sexiness, a warmth of character and a magnetic personality if the mount is well-developed, firm but springy to the touch. A tough cookie who holds everything in, if the mount is hard. Whereas softness here shows a receptive and sympathetic nature, a flabby consistency denotes a person who is lazy and self-centred.

When well-proportioned: Full of *joie de vivre*, loving, outgoing, exuberant are characteristic descriptions belonging to this type of development. Physically, these people tend to be energetic and robust and have the ability to simply shake off ill-health, whether of a physical or mental nature. A good libido accompanies this type of mount.

When over-developed: If the mount appears excessively large and disproportionate to the rest of the hand it denotes a hot-tempered and aggressive individual. The basic animal instincts prevail when this mount is developed to excess. When marked in this way, excessive sensuality, a huge appetite for personal and sexual gratification together with a need for over-stimulation of the senses is indicated. In some cases, sadistic tendencies might also be expected with this development, especially so if the rest of the palm feels hard as a board.

When thin and narrow: Mean, narrow-minded and selfish describes this character. There is a marked lack of energy and vitality with this development, an underactive metabolism being a possible underlying cause. Additionally, there could well be emotional difficulties for the owners of such a mount as this, accompanied by a poor sex drive. Here the problems could be physical, psychological or both.

- **Predisposition to ill-health:** Apart from a predisposition to sexually transmitted diseases amongst the more promiscuous of the sign, no particular tendencies are associated with Venusians. But it is fair to say that the fuller and more developed the mount, the more resistance there is to disease. The thinner and leaner the mount, the more the individual is vulnerable to ill-health and to whatever virus is currently doing the rounds. Indeed, the better constructed the mount, the healthier may be considered the individual and the stronger her vitality. Colour here may also be a clue to the general state of health of the individual although this must be judged firstly according to the prevailing ambient temperature and secondly in strict comparison to the rest of the hand. If the area is unduly pale or throws up an angry red colour, an imbalance of the metabolic processes may be suspected.

THE MOUNT OF LUNA

Your mount of Luna (from the Latin word for moon), anatomically known as your hypothenar eminence, is found on the opposite side to the thumb, low on the percussion edge just above the wrist. In some hands it may be developed outwards, thus forming a bow-window effect by pushing out the side of the palm, or alternatively it might be developed low down, forming a distinct knob just above the wrist. When this area looks heavy, thickly padded and overly full, as large as, or even larger than a normally developed Venus mount on its opposite side, it may be considered over-developed. When this part of the percussion edge of the palm is lean, shows little padding and lacks both breadth and height, it may be deemed as under-developed.

Physical characteristics: Constitutionally, Lunarians are not very strong and generally may be prone to ill-health.

Psychological profile: The Luna mount represents your sensitivity and intuition. A dreamy and romantic disposition, characteristic of the Luna influence, may at times develop into sentimentality and moodiness. Imagination, creativity and artistic ability is associated with this area. Sometimes when this mount is over-developed, the imagination can be allowed to run wild leading to mood swings, to depression and to states of hyperanxiety. Restlessness, coupled with mental and physical instability, mainly due to unrealistic expectations and to a sense of living with one's head in the clouds, is also represented here.

When well-proportioned: This is a sign of a sensitive, imaginative and creative mentality.

When over-developed: People possessing this development can all too easily construct their own reality for themselves, believing in their own delusions, suffering with too strong a 'Walter Mitty' streak in their character. These people are too impressionable for their own good. Renal and bladder disorders as well as rheumatic ailments are predispositions particularly associated with an over-large Luna mount. Neurosis, insanity and other afflictions of the mind are also linked with a large development here.

When thin and flat: A poorly developed – or even missing altogether – Luna mount denotes the valetudinarian, the hypochondriac who always fears something is wrong with his or her health.

• **Predisposition to ill-health:** Lunarians are prone to a wide range of problems including melancholia, moodiness, anxiety, restlessness and all manner of psychological disorders, especially so if the mount is much covered by many fine lines. Rheumatic ailments, problems of the bowels and large intestines, and gynaecological/urological problems are all associated with this type. So, too, is alcohol dependency (especially if the area is very red) and drug addiction (particularly emphasized by very white mounts). Lunarians are particularly vulnerable to both alcohol and drugs as these provide escapism from the harsh realities of life. 'Lunacy' and 'lunatic' are derived from the Latin word Luna as it was believed that the moon could cause madness and, interestingly, an excessively emphasized Luna mount is indeed associated with a predisposition to insanity and all manner of mental instability.

CENTRE PALM

The middle band of your palm incorporates the two mounts of Mars Positive and Mars Negative, found respectively on the thumb side and on the percussion edge. These two straddle the central area which isn't a mount at all but a comparatively flat stretch known as the plain of Mars. If the palm appears broader in the middle, or if this central band of your hand appears better developed than the top and basal parts, you are well equipped for handling physically or psychologically difficult conditions or stressful situations. Too broad, however, especially so on a very firm hand, can suggest aggressive tendencies.

Conversely, if this central band of your palm appears thin, narrow and poorly developed, heavily overhung by the mounts beneath your fingers and noticeably overshadowed by the mounts at your wrist, you are likely to suffer from a lack of resistance and you possess very little staying power. If this describes your hand, then you may not be so well equipped to deal with the stresses and strains of life and as such should seek a tranquil and harmonious environment in which to work and live. Peace, quiet, calm and serenity are essential to your health and well-being. On the negative side, you might lack a bit of moral fibre at times in that you tend to be too impressionable and all too easily distracted from your goals.

THE MOUNT OF MARS POSITIVE

The mount of Mars Positive is that fleshy pad that lies above the Venus mount and appears tucked under the wing of the thumb. When your thumb is held against the side of your hand and pressed into the edge of the palm, this mount forms a neat little hump. In those hands where it is large, hard in texture and causes the Life line to sweep out wide in order to accomodate it, the mount may be considered as disproportionately over-developed. Where there is hardly any development at all, such that there is either a dip or that the skin forms empty wrinkles when the thumb is pressed into the side of the palm, the mount may be judged to be deficient.

Physical characteristics: Generally of medium height, Martians tend to be strongly built, solid types often with powerful physiques. Healthwise, they enjoy a good, robust constitution and have plenty of energy and get-up-and-go.

Psychological profile: Courage, energy, a fighting spirit together with a sense of self-preservation and an ability to take charge and control of situations are the psychological qualities represented by this mount.

When well-proportioned: A courageous and healthy fighting spirit is denoted by a well-formed, well-proportioned Mars mount, one in which the owner is able to balance the principles of fight and flight.

When over-developed: When there is a disproportionately large development here there is a feeling of bottled-up aggression for this is very much the sign of the bully. Unless tempered by other factors, this large mount can be a beacon highlighting a dangerous personality. Brawn before brains tends to sum up the formation. In essence, and unless otherwise tempered, brute force, aggression and cruelty are the marks of a very large Mars mount. Owners of such developments seem to possess almost more physical energy than they know what to do with it. Often, then, it will spill out in the form of uncontrolled violence. Good advice for those with this formation who want to maintain a sense of well-being would be to learn to release their energies into physical training, on a sports field, perhaps, or through regular workouts in the gym. The adage 'A healthy mind in a healthy body' applies to these more than to any other type and should be seriously adopted as a way of life.

When thin and flat: Lack of positive drive, a tendency to be easily discouraged and give in, an inability to take control of their own lives, a weak nature and equally weak physical resources accompany a deficient mount here. These people easily tire themselves out and are ill-equipped to withstand the stresses and strains of modern life.

• **Predisposition to ill-health:** Feverishness, intestinal activity and bronchial conditions are associated with the Mars area. And because of the Martian hot temper and fiery disposition, cardiac problems are a particular weak link with this type. These predispositions are all the more emphasized if the mount is noticeably redder than its neighbours.

THE PLAIN OF MARS

The Plain of Mars is the central expanse of the palm that lies between the mounts of Mars Positive and Mars Negative.

Physical characteristics: The same kinds of physical character-istics are shared by all three Mars areas – a solid, well-built, overtly streetwise type of individual, someone who is strong and energetic.

Psychological profile: Self-control over one's passions and emotions is represented by this area of the palm.

When well-proportioned: When well-padded, this area denotes good powers of self-control, particularly control over one's emotions, aggression and reaction to life in general.

When over-developed: When too large in comparison to the rest of the hand, this formation suggests a sudden temper accompanied by flashes of uncontrollable rage. Desultory habits, drunkenness and lasciviousness may also be associated with this formation.

When thin: Poorly padded, so that the central palm appears thin and hollow, suggests a tendency to over-react to situations in life, especially so if this area is covered in fine, extraneous lines. To distinguish between a thin or a well-padded Plain of Mars, hold the palm between your thumb and fingers. If the tendons in the centre feel exposed and stringy, the area is thin. If they can't be felt, this area of the palm can be considered well-padded. A poor development here throws the spotlight on a weak character, someone who seems to lack any personal presence or sense of charisma and who doesn't possess the necessary stuffing to make a success out of life.

- **Predisposition to ill-health:** Similar indications as described above relating to the mount of Mars positive – prone to fevers, digestive, intestinal, bronchial and cardiac problems.

THE MOUNT OF MARS NEGATIVE

Your mount of Mars Negative is located on the percussion edge of the palm, opposite to your thumb. Because it is continuous with the Luna mount, the two are often indistinguishable from one another. If the mount is fleshy and well-developed it might push out the side of the palm to form a curved percussion edge.

Physical characteristics: Again, similar in stature to the other two types ruled by Mars – energetic, strong and robust both in body and in health.

Psychological profile: Self-control, moral resistance, staying power and the ability to cope when under pressure are represented by this mount.

When well-proportioned: Noticeable persistence and moral fortitude are qualities that go with this sort of development. When the mount appears harmoniously balanced with the rest, it denotes good moral fibre and integrity.

When over-developed: A disproportionately large mount here will show an individual who will doggedly stand firm when it comes to her beliefs and ideals regardless of whatever the evidence might show to the contrary. This is a person who, once she has made up her mind, cannot be persuaded against it – what might be called a truly 'bloody-minded' individual.

When thin and flat: A marked lack of resistance and moral fibre accompanies a poorly developed mount of Mars Negative.

- **Predisposition to ill-health:** Similar indications to the above two categories which denote feverishness, intestinal, bronchial and cardiac conditions.

Across the top of the palm lie four mounts, each forming the padding over the roots of the fingers and each taking its name from that of the finger above. Thus the first digit, also known as the finger of Jupiter, gives its name to the mount beneath which becomes the mount of Jupiter. Similarly, travelling across the top of the palm, the next area along is called the mount of Saturn, then comes the mount of Apollo and finally, reaching the other edge or percussion side of the hand, the mount of Mercury beneath the little finger.

THE MOUNT OF JUPITER
The mount of Jupiter is located at the top of your palm just beneath your index finger.

Physical characteristics: Jupiterian types are often well-built and, as a rule, they enjoy a robust and vigorous constitution.

Psychological profile: A personality that is warm and friendly, social and generous (with sometimes a tendency to extravagance) is the hallmark of the Jupiterian. If your mount is dominant, it is a sign that you are lively and noisy, and often seem able to fill a house all on your own. Characterized by your huge appetite, you are a lover of rich food and good wine and, unless there are signs denoting powers of restraint elsewhere in your hands, you consume plenty of both throughout your lifetime!

When well-proportioned: This shows a well-balanced and stable character, someone who is able to take things in her stride.

When over-developed: These are larger-than-life characters whose vast appetites could be the downfall of their health, especially so when the mount is not only over-developed but also very red in colour.

When thin and flat: Depression is a characteristic of an under-developed mount of Jupiter.

• **Predisposition to ill-health:** Because of their huge appetites and penchant for high living, most Jupiterians have a tendency to put on weight unless they are careful and watch their diets. Bronchial problems, intestinal complaints, hypertension and strokes are all diseases associated with the Jupiterian. Lines formed into long islands that lie across this mount may well confirm a vulnerability to chest infections and to coughs and colds in general.

THE MOUNT OF SATURN

The mount of Saturn is located at the top of your palm beneath your middle finger.

Physical characteristics: Often tall and thin with a prominent bone structure, Saturnians may be described as wiry types.

Psychological profile: Saturnians are typically sober-minded, serious, quiet, sensible types with plenty of self-control and who are readily able to shoulder responsibility. The negative side of the Saturnian produces introversion and such people seem to enjoy a morbid fascination in life. That is why many are characterized by their lugubriousness and fatalistic outlook.

When well-proportioned: Of all the mounts, this one should not be overly developed because when it is it denotes a morose individual, someone who is a loner and a misanthropist to boot. Better for this mount to be slightly on the flat side, neither over- nor under-developed. In comparison to its neighbours, the Saturn mount should always appear lower and flatter. When constructed in this way, it denotes good physical and mental health.

When over-developed: An over-developed mount here is the sign of an introverted personality with strong tendencies to paranoia, moodiness and depression. Such people find it difficult to express their affection for others and, because they are such critical nit-pickers, they may find that others are just as equally reluctant to give any affection back!

When thin and flat: General constitutional weaknesses accompany a very deficient Saturn mount. When noticeably under-developed there is a sense of irresponsibility and often a need for escapism.

• **Predisposition to ill-health:** Saturnians tend to lack vitality. Their teeth may be a source of trouble to them and, though many of the sign are musical, yet hearing problems are characteristic of this type. They are prone to biliousness, to nervous complaints, to rheumatic ailments in particular, to liver problems, varicose veins and haemorrhoids.

THE MOUNT OF APOLLO

The mount of Apollo is located at the top of your palm beneath your ring finger. It is not unusual to find that the development of this mount may be skewed slightly towards the little finger and merged with the Mercury mount. If these two mounts then appear to be the dominant ones in your hand, the qualities represented by each will be jointly manifested in your personality.

Physical characteristics: Typical Apollonians are of average stature but their bodies are graceful and agile with figures that might be described as athletic. As a rule they are very healthy types, undoubtedly due to the fact that they invariably take a happy and positive attitude to life.

Psychological profile: Positive, happy people with a lively and buoyant disposition. They are, as a rule, emotionally well-balanced people.

When well-proportioned: When of a good development there is a sunny disposition to the nature.

When over-developed: Extravagance, exhibitionism and vanity will be prominent features of the personality.

When thin and flat: Dull and emotionally repressed, these people have particular difficulty in communicating with others. Timidity and introversion will often hold them back in life. Heart trouble is one of the physiological weak links associated with flat Apollo mounts.

- **Predisposition to ill-health:** The cheerfulness and positive attitude of the Apollonian character seems to keep many of the usual maladies at bay. However, the diseases they are prone to include feverish conditions, problems with their sight and cardio-vascular diseases.

THE MOUNT OF MERCURY

The mount of Mercury is located at the top of your palm, directly beneath your little finger. In quite a few hands this area will be merged into the mount of Apollo and thus indistinguishable from it. Under these circumstances, an amalgamation of the qualities represented by both mounts will be pronounced in the character and personality of the individual concerned.

Physical characteristics: People with dominant Mercury mounts invariably have a Peter Pan quality about them that keeps them looking much younger than their years. Of medium to small stature, but all well-proportioned, the most telling characteristics of these types are their quick, nervous, almost bird-like gestures, their animated faces and their alert eyes that don't seem to miss a trick. In general, Mercurians enjoy fairly good health.

Psychological profile: The ability to communicate with others is represented by this mount. Well-padded and well-developed suggests a warm, receptive disposition, someone who is interested in the condition of others and in the affairs of the world. Poorly developed suggests a general lack of interest in other people and an inability to fully express oneself whether verbally, emotionally or sexually.

When well-proportioned: Socially well-balanced people who find it easy to integrate and communicate with others are denoted by this feature.

When over-developed: People whose Mercury mounts are disproportionately large tend to be the sort who live life in the fast lane and as such are prone to burnout. Thus, a tendency to nervous exhaustion is characterized by this formation. Additionally, because of their craving for constant excitement, such people may also be drawn to stimulants such as drugs and alcohol to provide the 'hit' or the 'charge' they feel is so essential to keeping their mood buoyant.

When thin and flat: Apathy is the characteristic trait most associated with a poorly formed mount here. Lisps, stammers and a variety of speech defects sometimes accompany a deficient mount of Mercury.

- **Predisposition to ill-health:** Nervous tension and stress are by far the biggest problems associated with this type. Intestinal or liver problems directly caused by anxiety are also a marked feature of the Mercurian disposition.

2

Health in our Hands

For centuries doctors have recognized the value of diagnostic clues that can be picked up from even the most perfunctory look at our hands. At a glance, our gestures will give the first tell-tale hints about how we are feeling. On closer examination, though, there's a good deal more specific information that can be gleaned from the hand about our physical state of health. The colour, the temperature and the general feel of our hands, can all help to clarify symptoms and can contribute towards a final diagnosis.

As long ago as the third century BC, Hippocrates, the father of medicine, observed that illnesses cause specific irregularities in the nails. Modern scientific research has indeed backed up his theories and has been able to show that the delicate growth process of the nail is sensitive to even the minutest physiological changes. Any hiccup, then, whether organic or nutritional, chronic or acute, will in some way register itself in the actual fabric of the nails. Abnormal growth, furrowing, pitting, splitting, or discolouration are some of the ways in which diseases, both of a temporary or long-term nature, will leave their marks.

In recent times, medical research has focused its attention on skin ridges and fingerprints in an attempt to match particular patterns to specific disorders. A great deal of work has been carried out in this field to date and the findings confirm a link between skin ridge patterns and genetic or chromosomal abnormalities. Though the most recognized and best documented correlation has been found between abnormal patterns and Down's Syndrome, studies involving other genetic conditions are continuing apace.

So, whether it is with a cursory glance or with a more in-depth

investigation, our hands do indeed seem to provide enormous
diagnostic material from which we can each begin to build a profile
of our health.

GESTURE

As soon as you step into the consulting room, an astute doctor will
immediately start to assess your psychological state of health simply
by looking at your body language. How you hold yourself, how you
walk, how you sit, will all give valuable clues about you and about
how you are feeling. And an important part of that assessment will
include how you use your hands: whether you hold them limply
or use animated gestures, whether you hold them in a relaxed pose
or make little nervous movements with them, whether they shake
or show signs of tremor. Most of the time, we use gesture without
even being aware of it. Our body language and our gestures are
part and parcel of the way we communicate with others because
communication isn't just a matter of expressing our thoughts in
words. With or without language we still transmit messages about
ourselves to other people – through the way we hold our bodies,
through our facial expressions, through the use of our hands and
our feet.

- Limply held hands convey a sense of dejection, of negativity.
  People who are dispirited and depressed, who feel they lack
  control over their lives, tend to just let their hands hang limply.
  It is a sign of a lack of spunk, little if no vitality, the stuffing
  seemingly to have been knocked out of these individuals.
  Physiologically, of course, those who are seriously ill might also
  let their hands and arms fall limply because they simply lack the
  physical strength to move their hands about in the normal way.
- Studies in a home for the mentally ill revealed some interesting
  insights into the way people hold their hands.
     The observations showed a tendency for the inmates to sit
  rocking themselves whilst holding their thumbs inside their
  clenched fists. Our thumbs, from the chirological point of view,
  are the most important of the digits as they represent our will-

power, our determination, our strength of character.

Hiding our thumbs, then, is a sign of withdrawal, it is tantamount to saying that we don't want to know, we don't want to exert our influence, we are either unwilling or incapable of using our will-power to change our circumstances.

- The way the thumb is generally held is altogether most insightful. One that is held rigidly close to the palm so as to form an acute angle betrays someone who is over-controlled. Those who are inhibited or who suffer from inner conflicts or tensions may display this sort of rigidity. A more flexible thumb, one which forms a wider angle to the rest of the hand, or whose tip has a supple bend, reveals a much more open and easy-going disposition.

- Perspiring is one of the autonomic responses to fear and because a vast number of sweat glands are particularly concentrated in the palm, we have all doubtlessly, at some time or other, experienced uncomfortably sweaty hands when we've been frightened or apprehensive. The most characteristic gesture that accompanies this is to wipe our hands down the sides of our thighs, or perhaps to wipe them with a hanky or a tissue.

- Jerky or rigid hand or arm movements are invariably a sign of tension and anxiety. So is fiddling. Drumming a tattoo on the table-top, fingers fussing over a button, or over the beads of a necklace, or twisting a strand of hair round and round an index finger – all of these are instantly recognizable signs of nervousness, of anxiety, of a lack of self-confidence or of impatience. Another well-known and very obvious sign of anxiety is hand-wringing.

- Nail-biting is associated with a sense of insecurity. Badly bitten nails in an adult are a classic symptom of an anxious disposition.

- Confidence and self-assurance is conveyed by easy, flowing, controlled movements, hands held calmly in a relaxed pose.

- Arms and hands that are held close to the body, tucked into pockets out of sight, are a sign of an introverted nature or a defensive attitude.

- In contrast, wide, expansive movements, arms that are flung outwards and away from the body are associated with a more extroverted personality.

- Gestures betraying anger and aggression are too numerous and too well-known to list but a few of the salient ones involve clenching the hand into a fist and thumping it on a table, stabbing the air with the index finger or curling the fingers stiffly into a claw-like pose.

HAND TREMORS

As mentioned above, nervousness may be conveyed through urgent little hand movements such as hand-wringing or incessant fiddling with a coat button or with a ring. These movements, however, are quite distinct from involuntary tremors which provide part of the diagnostic information on a variety of illnesses. And although indeed nervousness itself or simple fear can also produce such involuntary tremors at one end of the scale, at the other there are certain medical conditions known particularly to be associated with characteristic, and easily recognized, tremblings of the hand.

For instance, too many cocktails the night before may well produce, to the chagrin of the drinker, a shaky hand the following morning. Delirium tremens, or the DTs as they are more commonly called, following a wild night on Piña Coladas or Tequila Sunrises, should soon pass off the next day. But an inveterate drinker, though, will be given away by a constant fine tremor of the hand which will only be cured after the individual has 'dried out'.

The shakes, familiar consequence of an over-indulgence of alcohol, may equally occur as a result of drug abuse. But similar symptoms, too, may implicate toxicity in cases where the patient has swallowed large doses of certain minerals. Lead or mercury poisoning, for example, is often accompanied by a fine tremor of the hands.

In a case where hyperthyroidism is suspected, the doctor will ask the patient to hold out his or her arms and watch for any trembling of the fingers. With this hormonal disorder a fine tremor affecting the hand is one of its characteristic early symptoms, and the trembling is especially aggravated when the arm is extended and the fingers stretched out.

Still in the fine tremor category may be included symptoms which, when diagnosed correctly, can alert the doctor to disorders of the central nervous system or to diseases which progressively waste away the muscles. A more dramatic tremor may occur in multiple sclerosis. Here, the muscle spasms may produce a coarse shaking when the individual reaches out to touch an object, although no tremor exists when the hand is relaxed or at rest.

As with all aspects of health it is essential to stress time and again that diagnosis in hand analysis should never be attempted either from signs in the hands alone or, more generally, by anyone other than a qualified medical practitioner. Fine tremors are a case in point for they can easily be confused with other conditions, such as familial tremor, a harmless condition which is inherited, or with cases of hypoglycaemia (low glucose levels in the bloodstream). Even drinking too much strong coffee can bring on the shakes, albeit temporarily. And any of these may produce quite similar symptoms and cause great alarm if mistaken for the more serious disorders of the nervous system.

In the case of familial tremor, for example, this inherited condition is not associated with any particular disease but seems to occur when the individual is emotionally aroused or when particularly self-conscious. And although hypoglycaemia, or low blood sugar, is a condition more often associated with diabetes, it can and does occur more innocuously as a result of an over-strict dieting regime. Going without food for long periods of time may well induce a fine trembling in the fingers which then disappears when glucose or fruit juices are taken.

There is, however, one type of tremor that is unmistakable and is known as 'pill-rolling', an involuntary rhythmic movement of the thumbtip rubbing against the tip of the index finger. This specific tremor is a characteristic symptom of Parkinson's disease. The tremor symptomatic of this condition tends to occur when the hand is at rest, but disappears with movement.

THE COLOUR OF THE HAND

Just as with tremor, the actual colour of our hands, as well as any unnatural discolouration of the skin, can give obvious clues about our health. It can also reveal some of our habits!

One such is smoking where brown stains on the tops of the first two fingers invariably betray the heavy smoker. The attendant effects to one's health from this habit are too numerous to list here, but an investigation of the smoker's hand may well reveal whether other factors exist which could be aggravated by smoking. A predisposition to disorders of the respiratory tract, for example, is quite easy to spot and if the slightest susceptibility to chronic bronchitis, coronary disease or even cancer of the lungs is suspected then the message here is quite plain. Hand analysis teaches us that the colour of our hands reflects much about our character and disposition and, by association, identifies specific weak links in our health.

However, before formulating any conclusions about the colour of your skin, you *must* take into account the ambient temperature and, equally important, consider what activity has just taken place. A cold hand that's blue after an hour in a snow blizzard is not the same thing as a blue hand at room temperature! Nor should the warm beige of a skin that's been baked on the sands in Ibiza be confused with the yellowing more commonly associated with jaundice. And having just jogged a couple of times around the local football field may well cause your hands to go a healthy rose colour - quite a different thing to bright red hands when all you've been doing is sitting in front of the television all afternoon.

And whilst most of the information regarding health aspects in the hand is common to all nationalities, unhappily not enough research has been carried out on the colour changes in black hands. But since colour is only one factor which is taken in conjunction with many other features, there should, nevertheless, be enough clues elsewhere in the hand to arrive at a satisfactory conclusion across all races.

Hand Colour	Psychological Make-up	Health Indicators
Very red	Irascible temperament. Anger. Passion. Energy.	Possible high blood pressure. Possible liver dysfunction, especially cirrhosis of the liver. Glandular disorders. Gouty conditions.

Hand Colour	Psychological Make-up	Health Indicators
		Susceptibility to stroke. Diabetes. Feverish conditions. High temperatures. Exposure to chemicals, to allergens or to inclement weather conditions. Reddish blush on percussion sometimes a sign of pregnancy.
Pinkish	A well-balanced disposition.	Whatever the race, a pinkish tinge to the hand is the sign of a healthy constitution.
White	Self-centredness. Lack of warmth towards others. Lack of energy or enthusiasm.	Possible iron deficiency/anaemia. Poor circulation. Low blood pressure. Anxiety. Shock.
Blue or bluish grey		Circulatory, cardio-vascular or respiratory problems, especially if the hand is both blue and warm. Known as cyanosis, the condition can tinge with blue the nail-bed, nails and eventually affect the fingers and palms as well. Shock can turn hands blue but here the blueness will be accompanied by a cold and clammy feel to them. Adverse reactions to chemicals or drugs have been known to turn the skin and nail-beds bluish-grey. Effects from severe cold.

Hand Colour	Psychological Make-up	Health Indicators
Yellow		Jaundice. Severe cases of pernicious anaemia. Hepatitis. An excess of beta carotene (from eating a huge quantity of carrots or drinking too much carrot juice) can turn the skin yellow. If none of these conditions are corroborated, a yellow tinting of the skin can sometimes point to a very high cholesterol count, thus putting the cardio-vascular system in jeopardy.

Certain auto-immune disorders may also cause abnormal pigmentation of the skin on the hands. Vitiligo, for example, is a condition which produces pale patches of skin giving the hand a rather blotchy appearance, whilst in the condition known as Addison's disease the skin takes on a darker pigmentation, as if the hand were tanned although, of course, there has been no exposure to the sun or to artificial tanning agents.

TEMPERATURE

Variations of heat and cold, together with excessive moisture or dryness, are corroborative diagnostic signs of a variety of conditions and states of health.

Although the normal temperature may vary from one individual to another, the ideal healthy hand should not be too hot nor too cold, not too dry nor too moist. In certain cases, the temperature of the hand may give a good insight into the state of the endocrine, or glandular, system.

- Hands that are **too cold** despite a warm ambient temperature may well denote a circulatory problem.
- If the hands are **cold and dry** with a doughy feel to them, they could well suggest an underactive thyroid, particularly if the fingers are also podgy and remind you of sausages. Obesity would be another confirmatory symptom here.
- Shock, whether brought on by injury or sudden emotional trauma, produces characteristic physiological symptoms amongst which is a **cold, clammy** feel to the hands. This is often accompanied by excessive perspiration. But mild anxiety and nervousness can also make the hands go cold and sweaty.
- **Hot, sweaty** hands (whose owner hasn't just been doing aerobics!) may be a corroborating symptom of an overactive thyroid.
- Hands that are **hot and dry** may be associated with hypertension. This can also be a symptom of kidney problems.
- **Very hot and dry** hands often accompany a high fever.
- A **warm, dry** skin, unless otherwise dried through overuse of detergents, chemicals or solvents, could be symptomatic of nutritional deficiencies.

THE NAILS

For centuries, fingernails have been used as diagnostic clues to health disorders. As far back as 400 BC, Hippocrates recognized the value of the shape and development of the nails in reflecting disease. Indeed, a particular type of nail, attributed to his own findings, which reflects certain respiratory disorders, is still widely recognized today. So it is that the **Hippocratic nail** has been named, as its title implies, after the venerable physician himself.

Even in today's modern surgery our fingernails can be a valuable source of information when it comes to our state of health and well-being. As already mentioned, merely at a glance badly chewed nails will suggest a nervous disposition, and brown stained indices may well give away a heavy smoker. But still closer investigation will reveal far more important insights into the organic workings of the body. Here may be found some pretty impressive clues as to the cardio-vascular system, glandular functioning, nutritional balance as well as all manner of infection and disease, that might afflict us physiologically as well as psychologically.

It is essentially because of its sensitivity and response to the underlying blood supply that the condition of the nail itself is a good register upon which signs of disease are imprinted. If the blood supply is deficient in any way it will instantly have a bearing on the growth of the nail itself. Both injury and illness, then, may result in abnormal development, deformities and discolouration of our fingernails.

Nails are made of a protein material called **keratin**, a substance that is found throughout the animal kingdom and that produces hair, claws, feathers, and surprisingly enough, hooves and such things as the rhino's horn as well. Essentially, the function of the nail is primarily a protective one for it guards the nerve-rich, sensitive tip of the finger against injury. As an evolution from claws, its secondary function may be said to be that of defence – a well-sharpened nail can inflict a good bit of damage in a carefully aimed swipe. But in grooming the body, most especially, nails play an essential part. Imagine just for a moment the sheer bliss of scratching an irritating itch with your fingernails! Equally, if it weren't for our fingernails, everyday manipulative actions such as picking up small objects, for example, or carrying out minute tasks with our fingers would be made that much more difficult.

The manufacture of the nail is an ongoing process, each nail taking roughly six months to grow from cuticle to quick, that is, to the end of the pink 'living' part of the nail. The free edge, or white tip, is that part which grows out from the 'matrix', or nail bed, and once detached from the living cells may then be cut or manicured according to the lifestyle demands of the individual. In all assessments of the nails, whether of the shape or size, it is to the quick, or the pink living part, and not to the white tip that the information applies.

Interestingly, though on average our fingernails take something between 160 and 180 days to develop, the actual growth rate differs according to our age and health, according to the season, to whether they are our fingernails or our toenails, to whether they are on our right or left hands, and even according to the very digit the nail is on.

For a start, our toenails grow at a quarter the rate of our fingernails, so that the nails on our thumbs will grow as much in one week as the nails on our big toes do in one month. When we are young our nails grow faster than when we are old. In the warmer weather of summertime they put on a greater spurt than they do in the winter. Right-handers amongst us will find that they have to file down the nails on their right hands more frequently than those on their left (vice versa for left-handers). And even our middle and index fingernails seem to outpace those on our ring and little fingers, though it's our thumbnails that grow faster than all the rest.

Production of the nail takes place below the surface of the finger some three-quarters of a centimetre beyond the cuticle. Gently press the base of your thumbnail and you will notice a corresponding slight depression in the finger where the nail plate continues towards its root. Here, at its point of inception, the nail begins to be formed in a perpetual on-going process, soft and gel-like at first, then hardening into compressed layers as it pushes its way out, conveyor-belt style, over the end of the digit.

Around its edge, each nail is protected by a flap of skin called the cuticle which acts as an airtight shield against dirt and infection that might invade and endanger the delicate growth mechanism beneath. The semi-circular moon, or lunule, at its base is part of the dense growing root and shows up as milky-white. Moons are more commonly seen on thumbs and less frequently so on the little fingers. Size and colour of the lunule add to the diagnostic properties of the nail.

As the nail grows out over the nail-bed, the horny layers become transparent and the familiar pinkiness associated with nails is not, in fact, due to the fabric of the nail itself but to the blood-rich capillaries in the nail-bed that feed and nourish the nail above. For Hippocrates, this was the window to the condition of the individual's health, for the colour here would give invaluable clues to the nature of the humours. Too red, for example, suggested to him a dangerously choleric disposition, whilst too white might display signs of a phlegmatic constitution. And just as in his day, the colouration of our nails can even now play an important diagnostic role in the modern GP's surgery.

It is precisely because the nails are continually being made, night and day, hour after hour, that they respond so instantly to any hiccups in their growth process. Any interruption to the blood supply, poor diet, or a sudden shock which rocks the nervous system will each affect the delicate growth mechanism and register its complaint either in the actual fabric and composition of the nail itself or in the pigmentation of the bed beneath.

Indeed, it is good nutrition, obtained from a varied, balanced diet, which is not only fundamental in providing optimum health but which is also essential to the healthy growth of the nail. Poor nutrition, especially, sends ripples throughout our systems, any deficiencies particularly registering themselves in the nails in a variety of ways, in the form of horizontal grooves, for example, amongst other markings.

Grabbing a sandwich as you rush off to those important meetings each afternoon, living off chips and processed food or alternatively deciding to go on a sudden crash diet may all leave their imprint in the form of these horizontal ridges across your nails. These grooves, known as 'Beau's lines', are of particular interest for two fundamental reasons. Firstly, they confirm the growth rate of the nail. And secondly, their appearance, coinciding with injury or trauma to the system (whether of a physical or psychological nature) corroborates the fact that a catastrophic event disrupts the smooth flow of the keratinous material that makes up the nail.

So, unless a groove is stamped in through a direct injury to the nail itself, it is formed at its root, or growing point, and then progresses upwards as the nail grows out. And because it is known that a nail takes approximately six months to grow from root to tip, it is possible then to make a rough estimate of when that particular injury or trauma too place.

A horizontal groove occurring half-way up your nail, for example, would suggest that you went on a crash diet, or perhaps suffered a shock of some sort, roughly three months ago. Lower down, a groove would point to the incident having taken place more recently, perhaps only a month or two in the past. And, similarly, higher up would point to the event having occurred around five to six months previously. And of course, as with all diseases represented either by discolouration or irregularities of the nails, once recovery takes place the nails return to normal.

Vitamins A and **D** are believed to be helpful in maintaining

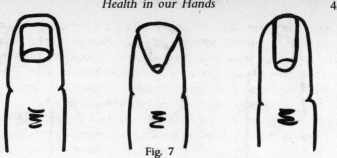

Fig. 7

healthy nails, as are **Silica** amongst the tissue salts, as well as **Combination K** which is specially recommended for brittle nails and falling hair.

Apart from the physiological aspects, on the psychological side, too, it has been recognized over the centuries that the shape of our nails reflects our temperament. And it is that temperament that describes our physical constitution, that colours our view of life, governs our interaction with others, affects how we deal with events and circumstances and generally highlights our mental and emotional well-being.

Broadly speaking, shapes may be broken into three main categories – the square, the fan shape and the long, though each category may be subdivided still further. The three different types of nails may be seen in Figure 7. Whilst the size of the nail must be viewed in relation to the size of the hand itself, a general rule to bear in mind when correlating nail shape to temperament is that the smaller the nail, the more critical the individual and the more narrow that person's point of view and outlook on life. People with small nails have a greater tendency towards cardio-vascular problems, especially so from middle age on. The larger the nail, the more even-tempered will be the individual and the more placid and broad-minded the nature. Health problems with this type may tend towards the nervous or psychological disorders.

THE SQUARE NAIL

- Characterized by parallel sides and a straight base. This type of nail shows a stable temperament, someone who is fairly

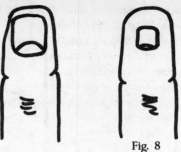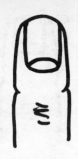

Fig. 8

equanimical and slow to anger. Owners of this type take a rather sanguine view of life; they tend to be more the hale and hearty type.

- When the square nail is very short it reflects a nervous, critical, irritable nature, prone to emotional affectation and neurosis. People possessing such nails tend to be selfish and noticeably lacking in warmth towards others.
- The longer variation in this category, which is more rectangular in shape, reflects a much more even-tempered individual, someone who is slow to anger. There is a certain fussiness or meticulousness about this type of person which, when it comes to matters of health, may incline the subject towards a touch of hypochondria.

THE WIDE NAIL

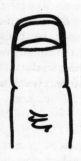

Fig. 9

- Characterized by a straight base and parallel sides but this nail is much broader in comparison to its height.
- Psychologically, the wide nail reflects a quick temper that wells up suddenly like a volcano but which, once exploded, subsides leaving no lasting sulkiness or recriminations.
- Physiologically, those possessing this type of nail are considered constitutionally strong and resilient although some chirologists describe this as an apoplectic type.

THE FAN-SHAPED NAIL

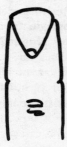

Fig. 10

- Characterized by a triangular shape where the nail tapers to a point at its root.
- This is a sign of an emotionally sensitive and highly-strung disposition.
- Psychologically, people possessing such nails tend to act on impulse and may show signs of irrational or neurotic behaviour.
- Physiologically, nails may adopt this shape as a result of severe stress or following emotional shock. Indeed, when this shaped nail is present it is an important warning sign that stress is one of the weak links which could easily undermine the owner's health, the nervous system being especially under seige.

THE LONG, NARROW NAIL

- Characterized by a rounded base and narrow enough to display a good deal of digit either side of the nail.
- With a full set of long, narrow nails there is emotional instability.

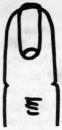

Fig. 11

Individuals with this type of nail may also be fairly repressed
and prone to psychological disorders.

- Physiologically, these people do not enjoy robust health and may
  generally be considered physically delicate. They possess,
  however, a great deal of nervous energy.
- Nails that are extremely narrow highlight hypersensitivity.
- Those that are narrow and thick, with a tendency to curve into
  a talon shape, suggest dietary deficiencies coupled with poor
  elimination.

Any deformities of the actual horny layer, any distortions or
abnormal construction of the nail itself point to damage of the
actual growth process. As such, these irregularities are associated
with particular malfunction, with injury to the system and with a
variety of physiological disorders.

THE CONCAVE NAIL

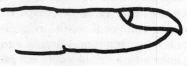

Fig. 12

- Characterized by a pronounced dished or spooned appearance.
- Generally, a lack of energy and a lacklustre vitality accompanies
  a full set of dished nails.
- Constant exposure to chemicals, to water or to certain softeners
  such as oils, for example, may swell and soften the nails to such

an extent that they curve upwards as they grow and become characteristically spoon-shaped.

- Occasionally the condition is found in the hands of individuals suffering certain mental illnesses.
- Physiologically and more typically, the concave nail is a sign of dietary or nutritional deficiencies where a serious mineral imbalance occurs, thus weakening and thinning the very fabric of the nail itself. Recovery follows improved diet together with vitamin, mineral or tissue salt supplements.
- The concave nail is also associated with iron deficiency anaemia. It is fairly common amongst women both of child-bearing and pre-menopausal age but the nails respond well to treatment and usually return to normal when iron supplements are taken. Otherwise, the concave nail is also associated with certain skin disorders, with underactivity of the thyroid gland and with some types of venereal disease.

THE CONVEX NAIL

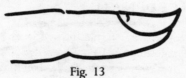

Fig. 13

- Characterized by a marked curvature of the nail whereby the tip of the nail wraps itself over and around the tip of the finger.
- This feature often points to respiratory problems and may be found in the hands of smokers. Interestingly, the curving follows a discreet pattern with the nail on the left index finger being the first to curve. This is followed by the nail on the right index and subsequently by the left middle finger, followed by the right middle finger. Persistent coughs, colds and bronchitis often accompany the condition thus emphasizing the onslaught upon the lungs and bronchi. Progressive weakening of the lungs will be reflected by all ten nails hooked over the tips of the fingers. However, when the individual gives up smoking the improvement of the respiratory system will be reflected by the fact that the nails return to normal.

Some hand analysts have suggested that it takes about two

years to right this condition after the individual has stopped smoking. But here I feel compelled to add a personal note, for I used to be a heavy smoker myself, and I watched this curious phenomenon, with great interest and not a little alarm, taking place in my own hands. Sure enough the distortion began on my left index and then on my right. After some months I noticed that the two middle nails had followed suit and all four were so tightly hooked around my fingertips that it became impossible to pick up coins lying on a table-top. Instead, I had to slide them to the edge and let them drop into my hand. Fortunately, before the degeneration spread to the nails on my ring fingers and beyond, I saw the light and gave up smoking. But it took some five to six years or so for my nails to return to normal and throughout that time I personally found the tissue salts Silica and Combination K, both recommended for weak and brittle nails, of great benefit in restoring my nails back to their former state.

THE HUMPED NAIL

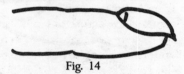

Fig. 14

- A more serious condition than the curved nail because, whereas with the former it is only the tip that curves over, here the tissues of the nail-bed become swollen so that the whole nail humps or rises upwards from the cuticle, giving the whole nail a rather bulbous look.
- Sometimes called the Hippocratic nail, after Hippocrates who first described it and associated it with such lung diseases as pneumonia and tuberculosis, it is still recognized today as a symptom of certain respiratory disorders. A predisposition to cardio-vascular problems, to emphysema and heart disease is also associated with the humped nail. In addition, it can also be symptomatic of cirrhosis of the liver. This malformation is recognized in severe cases, where the fingers also show signs of clubbing (i.e. distort and grow bulbous at their tips) together with other signs such as cyanosis, or a blue discolouration,

as amongst the symptoms of lung tumours. On its own, however, the Hippocratic nail can reflect poor oxygenation and, like the former curved nail, will return to normal when the condition has responded to treatment.

HORIZONTAL RIDGING

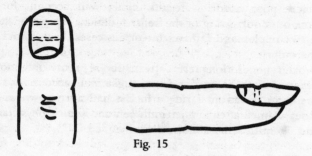

Fig. 15

- Characterized by horizontal dents or grooves in the nails, sometimes occurring singly and sometimes forming a series of corrugations from cuticle to tip.
- A single horizontal ridge across one nail is almost certainly a result of damage or injury to that nail. When a horizontal ridge is seen on all the nails it could well be registering a shock to the system. The trauma implied could either be physical or psychological in origin. Because the nails take on average six months to grow from cuticle to tip, it is possible to calculate when the trauma occurred. Close to the base would suggest a recent shock, half-way up the nail records that the event took place something like three months ago, and further up near the tip would suggest the onslaught occurred some five or six months previously. A sudden crash diet, a short burst of acute stress or an emotional upset, such as an unexpected bereavement perhaps, might account for such a marking in the nail.
- The sudden interruption to the blood supply, as might occur in the case of a heart attack, would also interfere with the normal production of the nail and thus leave its characteristic marking in this form.
- Infectious diseases, too, such as mumps or measles, could well

be responsible for the appearance of horizontal indentations across the nails.

- High fevers have been known to mark their occurrence in this way.

- If all the nails show a series of horizontal ridges they represent a longer period of disturbance to the system. Serious dieting, where poor nutrition results, could well account for such horizontal furrowing of the nails. A deficiency of the Vitamins A, B-complex and D have, in certain cases, been found to be the culprit.

- Broken bones, long-term stress, severe acute infections or illnesses such as scarlet fever might well account for these markings. Horizontal ridges in the nail are known as **Beau lines**, named after a nineteenth century French physician who first identified the abnormality.

VERTICAL RIDGING

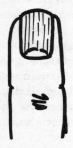

Fig. 16

- Characterized by ribs within the very fabric of the nail itself which feel bumpy when you run your thumbnail across them. These ridges are also caused by irregular production of the nail tissue, and whilst one might assume that the ribbing acts as reinforcement, the contrary seems to be the case: that, in actual fact, their appearance denotes brittleness.

- Heavy vertical ridging tends to occur more frequently with age but can be associated with a delicate physiological system that is sensitive to certain allergens.

- In many cases, nails that are ridged in this way are considered

to be hereditary and as such will highlight inherited susceptibilities such as, for example, a predisposition to gout or other rheumatic conditions. Rheumatoid arthritis is especially linked to a full set of nails that are heavily ridged in this way.
- It is also believed that an overactive thyroid gland may be responsible for laying down these thickened ribs in the nail.
- Some chronic skin diseases as well as certain gastric disorders, too, are linked with ridged nails.

PITTING

- Tiny indentations reminiscent of pin-pricks may suggest the onset of psoriasis. Other diseases affecting the auto-immune system might also be implicated by severe pitting of the nails.

THICKENING OF THE NAIL

- In cases where the nails start to thicken and toughen noticeably, becoming hard to cut, and especially if they also take on a yellow hue, problems of the lymphatic system, cardio-vascular diseases or diabetes may be implicated.
- Amongst the disorders affecting the skin which also leaves its mark on the nails is psoriasis. In severe cases this condition may cause the nails to thicken and detach themselves from the nail bed. In less extreme cases the nails become roughened with characteristic indentations pitting the surface.

BRITTLE NAILS

- Thin, flaky or brittle nails can be a sign of a mineral imbalance. However, it must always be borne in mind that this type of nail may be caused by environmental conditions. Constant exposure to water, to oils or to chemicals can adversely affect the nails, leaving them weak and prone to splitting.
- A lack of calcium and protein may be responsible for weak, soft nails.
- Brittle nails that are slow to grow and that lack lustre may also be associated with hypothyroidism, otherwise known as an underactive thyroid gland.

WEATHER EFFECTS ON THE NAILS

- Cold, damp weather may affect the nails, causing them to soften and weaken.
- In winter, the nails tend to grow more slowly than they do in the summer and are also more prone to breaking in the cold weather.
- In particularly damp parts of the country, nails may absorb a good deal of moisture. This can result in softening, flaking or even, in severe cases, of actual distortion of the shape of the nail itself.

THE MOONS

- Like so many other features of the hand, the type, shape and colour of the moons may well be inherited and thus bring along with them any familial predisposition to disease that is genetically inherent.
- Ideally, the moons should be milky-white in colour.
- Most commonly, moons are seen on the thumbs and less rarely on the little fingers. In fact, in many hands only the moons on the thumbs are visible, the rest being hidden beneath the skin.
- Over-large moons suggest a predisposition to an overactive thyroid.
- No moons at all may suggest an underactive thyroid gland. In general, a weaker constitution is associated with moonless nails.
- Poorly formed moons may point to a predisposition to heart disease.
- Moons that are tinged with blue denote respiratory disorders and possible cardio-vascular problems.

COLOUR OF THE NAILS

In the ideal hand, the colour of the nail-bed should match the pigmentation of the palm, so that in the European hand the nail has a healthy pinkish tinge to it, whilst in the African hand the nail tends to be of a pinky-beige hue. Smooth, transparent and with a satiny sheen, it should be gently rounded from side to side and slightly springy from top to bottom. Moons should be well defined and milky-white in colour.

Just as with the pigmentation of the skin, the colour of the nail bed which shows through the horny layer that constitutes the nail reflects the state of the vascular system.

- Too pallid can be a sign of iron-deficiency anaemia. A lack of energy and a general low vitality is associated with nails that are very pale pink in colour.
- White, and sometimes even yellow, can point to liver dysfunction. Certain venereal diseases, too, are associated with whitish-yellow nail-beds.
- Cyanosis, caused by circulatory problems such as occurs with a deoxygenated blood supply, leaves its characteristic blue tinge within the nail-bed.
- Yellow nails can suggest jaundice and other problems affecting the liver. A surfeit of beta carotene, however, will also leave a distinctive yellow tinge on the nail-beds.
- Very red suggests high blood pressure and a tendency towards cardio-vascular diseases. An irascible temperament also goes with red nails.

Other than the uniform discolouration of the nail bed, a variety of coloured speckling may also occur.

SPECKS, SPOTS AND OTHER COLOURED MARKINGS

- White spots or specks in the nail have long been considered a sign of calcium deficiency, in particular that of calcium phosphate. This may indeed be the case but as many people with these markings have not found an improvement when augmenting their intake of calcium-rich foods, it would suggest that perhaps another agent is either deficient or at fault, and thus impeding adequate assimilation of the mineral. Current thinking lays the blame on a deficiency of zinc, magnesium and possibly, too, on a deficiency of the vitamin B6.
- On the psychological side, tiredness and anxiety can produce these characteristic speckled marks, too. Interestingly, the speckling disappears as the stress levels are reduced and the problems are resolved.

- Horizontal white lines which occur in the nail but which do not cause the fabric of the nail itself to actually form into ridges, as in the Beau's lines, are known as **Mee's lines**. Whilst in some cases these lines denote nutritional deficiencies, they are more widely documented as reflecting poisoning from certain minerals such as arsenic and thallium. They are particularly associated with acute fever and also implicated in certain coronary diseases.

- One of the symptoms of bacterial infection of the valves of the heart is recognized as tiny bruises that show up in the form of long, thin black specks underneath the nail.

- Similar streaks, but this time red in colour, are associated with long-term high blood pressure. Bacterial infection of the heart may be implicated in severe cases.

- When the nail bed is pale in colour with a thin red band appearing towards the top near the free edge of the nail, liver disease may be suspected.

- Nails where the basal half are a brownish-fawn colour whilst the top half are white are associated with renal disease.

But of course, apart from reflecting the mental and physical state of the individual's health, the nail itself may come under attack from a variety of disorders mainly involving bacterial or fungal infection. One of the most common of these is **paronychia**, a condition which causes the nail-bed, the cuticle and the surrounding fingertip to swell and become very sore indeed. If not treated, the condition results in damage to the nail, thickening, severe ridging, discolouration and eventual distortion.

PAPILLARY RIDGES

Papillary ridges are formed as part of the top layer of the skin that covers the palms of our hands and the soles of our feet and are more commonly recognized when they form themselves into patterns that make up our fingerprints. A closer study of the hand, however, will reveal that the ridges not only form themselves into patterns on the tips of our fingers but at various places on our palms as well.

Just as the nails give tell-tale clues about our current state of health and our predisposition to disease, so, too, the condition, formation and location of the papillary ridge patterns can give invaluable information about our individual pathology. And, just as with the nails, information gleaned from these patterns should never be used *on their own* as a means of diagnosis but should be used only as a tool in conjunction with other clinical parameters to confirm or lend weight to an already suspected diagnosis.

Incidentally, in scientific circles, this system of ridges is called dermatoglyphics - 'derma', meaning skin and 'glyph', a carving. Thus, the word dermatoglyphics neatly describes the ridges and furrows seemingly carved into the surface of the unique type of skin that covers our palms and, of course, the soles of our feet too.

Looked at in close-up, the ridging might be described as resembling sheets of corrugated iron with lines and furrows running parallel to each other but then, here and there, the corrugations swirl themselves into the complex patterns of loops, whorls and arches that are characteristically found on the tips of our fingers, at various other locations in the palm and on the soles and toes of our feet. It is from these patterns that measurements of the ridges are made and from which a classification system has been evolved.

Loops, whorls and arches are the three main categories of fingerprint patterns although two further types derived from these - the tented arch and the composite - may be added to bring the total classification to five. Years of matching patterns to their respective owners have brought to light distinctive personality characteristics associated with each category. On a psychological level, of course, these character traits will have a direct bearing on the mental and physical state of the individual's health.

When it comes to making any observations or taking measurements of skin patterns and fingerprints, it is essential to work in good light and preferably to view the hand under a magnifying glass. Except when taking just a cursory glance, it will be found easier to work from a print. Instructions on taking handprints are given in the Appendix.

THE LOOP

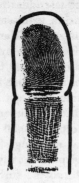

Fig. 17

- Flexible, versatile and adaptable, a majority of loop patterns is the sign of a co-operative nature and an easygoing disposition. These people especially enjoy masses of interests and a busy life, filled with plenty of variety. Quick to respond and react, they particularly enjoy the adrenalin surge that goes with an active and buzzing working and domestic lifestyle.
- Because of the personality generally associated with the loop pattern, susceptibility to nervous problems, such as nervous fatigue and even mental breakdown, may be suspected.

THE WHORL

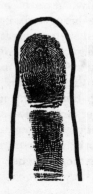

Fig. 18

- A majority of whorl patterns is the mark of intensity. Such people are deep thinkers, slow to respond and react and extremely individualistic in their tastes, opinions and philosophies in life. These are people who tend to keep their feelings to themselves.
- Inner tension which can lead to either intestinal, digestive or cardio-vascular problems is associated with this pattern and owners of whorls would do well to practise deep breathing relaxation techniques on a regular basis.

THE ARCH

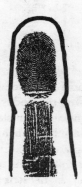

Fig. 19

- A majority of arch patterns will normally denote a practical, hard-working and down-to-earth individual. These people tend to possess a certain reserve in their nature which hinders their ability to verbalize their innermost feelings. This inarticulacy leads many possessing the arched fingerprints to repress their emotions.
- The tendency to bottle up their feelings and emotions can lead to ulcers and digestive disorders, on the physical side, and in extreme cases on the psychological side, to nervous breakdown.
- A predisposition to hypertension and inherited heart problems are associated with the arch pattern.
- Any form of creative pursuit which allows the free expression of their imagination is excellent cathartic therapy for the arched types. Any creative aptitude or leanings that might appear should be encouraged even from a very young age.

THE TENTED ARCH

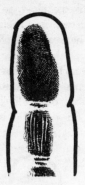

Fig. 20

- It is rare to find a whole set of tented arches. In general, these tend to occur only on the index or middle fingers. When present, they highlight an enthusiastic nature, someone who constantly needs to have his or her imagination fired with new projects and interests.
- Temperamentally sensitive, people possessing tented arches may show signs of being highly-strung and prone to nervous problems.
- Impulsiveness, which is a characteristic of this type, can lead to accidents and injury.

THE COMPOSITE

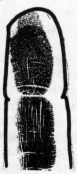

Fig. 21

- Just as with the tented arch, it is rare to find a complete set of composite patterns. When this fingerprint is present it will more usually be found on the thumbs and indices. Composite patterns show an inability to make up one's mind but a mentality which needs to see all sides of the picture, to weigh up all the pros and cons before reaching a conclusion.
- Mental fatigue can result from over-speculation and excessive brooding.

Though more generally associated with the tips of the fingers, similar patterns that make up the fingerprints may also be found on other parts of the palm as well. The 'open-field' arrangement of the skin ridges is the more commonly found on the thenar and hypothenar areas, or mounts of Venus and Luna, in the normal hand. This, as shown in Figure 22, is a free flow of the the ridge and furrow system, undisturbed by the more complex swirls of the loop and whorl patterns.

However, loops, whorls and arches do occur both on these areas and also on the palm just below the base of the digits. But of greater interest, and more important bearing on the question of health, are the patterns that occur on the Luna mount, or hypothenar, as these may reflect an above-average tendency to mental disorders. Under normal circumstances, a tendency or susceptibility is all that is implied and such markings are in no way absolute signs of mental disturbance. In the abnormal hand, though, research has shown that an increased incidence of complex patterns on the Luna area does seem to occur.

Earlier this century, much attention was focused on the papillary or skin ridges in an attempt, by medical researchers, to determine whether mental or physiological abnormalities imprint themselves in characteristic patterns on our palms and fingertips. From their studies, evidence was found to confirm that abnormal patterns in the skin ridges highlight a predisposition to certain types of mental illnesses. Further, it was shown that particular patterns may also point to various congenital and psychological disorders such as heart disease, for example, and obsessive or compulsive behaviour.

Apart from the more familiar configurations of loop, arch, and whorl, other patterns known as triradii, also present in the hand,

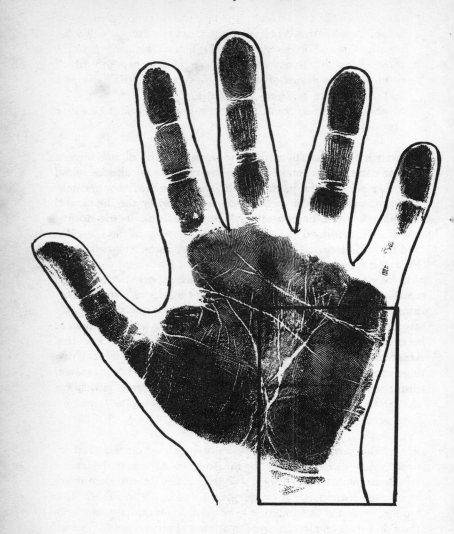

Fig. 22

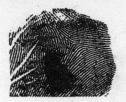

Fig. 23

play an important part in medical investigation. Triradii, illustrated in Figure 23, occur when three sets of ridges meet and form themselves into a triangular pattern more clearly seen at the top of the palm just beneath the fingers. One of the most important triangular formation of ridges may be seen at the base of the palm just above the wrist.

Both for forensic and medical purposes it is necessary to measure the size and quantity of ridges that constitute a fingerprint. Such measurements are achieved by drawing a line from the apex of the triradius to the central core of the skin pattern and counting the ridges in between (see Figure 24). This is known as the 'ridge count' which, in forensic analysis, is used to make an absolute match between latent prints collected at scenes of crime and the suspected criminal's own fingerprints. In medical research, the ridge count is a critical factor taken into account when comparisons are made between normal and abnormal hands.

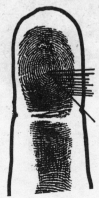

Fig. 24

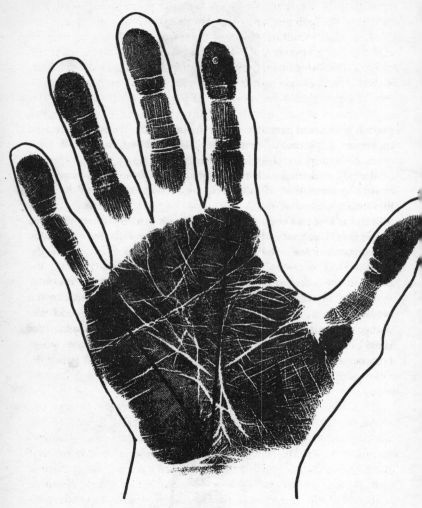

Fig. 25

In dermatoglyphic studies, particular attention is focused on three triradii, the first two located on the palm just beneath the index and little finger and named respectively 'a' and 'd', and the third, or axial triradius, which, in the normal hand, lies at the base of the palm, is known as 't'. When lines are drawn down from the two top triangular formations to join the third triradius at the base of the palm, the angle formed is known as the 'atd' angle, see Figure 25. Why this should be important is that in the normal hand the angle formed should measure roughly 45 degrees. If, however, the angle is much wider, due to the fact that the basal triradius occurs higher up in the palm, as in Figure 26, then studies suggest that some type of physical abnormality may exist.

All of these dermal patterns are genetically inherited and already formed by the fourth month of foetal development. Any inherited abnormality, chromosomal aberration or serious hiccough in the developmental process at that time will distort the papillary ridging and imprint itself in the form of abnormal patterns both in the palm of the hand and on the soles of the feet.

The results of the medical research, then, tend to substantiate the argument that people are predisposed to certain illnesses, regardless of environmental factors, lifestyle, conditioning or whatever. And, unlike the flexure lines, these markings do not change throughout one's lifetime. However, environmental factors, lifestyle and conditioning certainly *do* play a significant role when it comes to whether those predispositions ever develop into full-blown clinical diseases or simply remain latent at the blueprint stage.

So it is that genetic malformations which are handed down from parent to child will stamp themselves, in the form of abnormal skin markings, into the hand of the unborn infant. But so, too, can any trauma that directly affects the foetus, such as a disease or viral infection which the mother might contract during those critical early months of pregnancy. For example, babies whose mothers contract rubella, or German measles, during the first month or so of gestation, run over a 50 per cent risk of being born with major defects, and the skin markings in their hands will reflect those abnormalities.

Of all the research carried out in this field, the most conclusive results, and the most widely recognized, are the findings

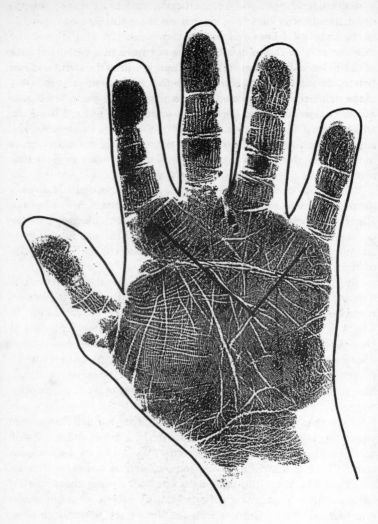

Fig. 26

concerning Down's Syndrome, otherwise known as mongolism, a condition directly caused by chromosomal abnormalities. Figure 27 is the print of a Down's Syndrome sufferer.

In the case of Down's Syndrome, apart from irregularities of the major lines, there are several features concerning the dermal ridges which, depending on the gravity of the condition, may recur. For example, the ridges tend to flow in a more horizontal direction across the palm due to the displacement further up in the hand

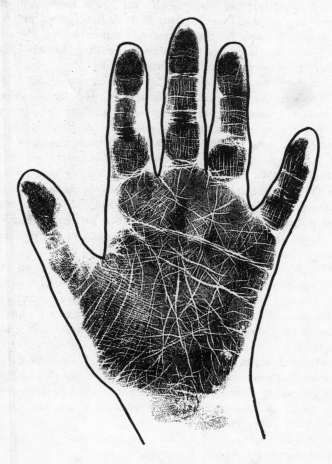

Fig. 27

of the axial triradius – the 'atd' angle being greater than 45 degrees. There is also a higher incidence of ulna loops on the fingertips and a greater likelihood of complex patterns occurring on the Luna mount, whilst a decrease of patterns in the Venus area has been observed.

Scientific studies have shown that either one or both parents of Down's Syndrome children themselves possess unusual ridge-patterns in their own hands. But though the parents may not show outward symptoms of mongolism, yet their dermatoglyphic patterns suggest that there is some fault in their genes and that this fault could well be transmitted to their offspring. Here, in particular, when it comes to genetic counselling, knowledge of papillary ridging could prove invaluable.

Although the wealth of research that has been carried out in this area confirms that almost all individuals with chromosomal abnormalities possess abnormal or unusual papillary ridge-patterns, it is not the case that different disorders mark the hand in characteristic ways specific only to each of those conditions. In short, it is not necessarily possible to distinguish one disorder from another simply by looking at the abnormal ridging in the hand. Nevertheless, aberrant patterns, whether because of their frequency, displacement or unusual formation, do seem to point to the possibility of some sort of physical or mental impairment due to any abnormalities that may be stamped in during foetal development.

Although, of course, there are wide variations in the dermatoglyphic patterns of what may be considered the *normal* hand, research has been able to show the types of patterns, or combination of factors, which do tend to recur more frequently in the average population. Marked deviation from the norm, though not 100 per cent confirming abnormality, would nevertheless point to the possibility of some kind of genetic defect. However, it is stressed once again that diagnosis of disease from ridge patterning alone is not reliable and should be considered solely as an aid in corroborating conditions which are already suspected by other symptoms.

Below is a comparison of the dermatoglyphic factors commonly associated with the typical and atypical hands:

The Typical Hand

The most common fingerprint pattern is the loop, closely followed by the whorl. Although of course they do occur, arches are less commonly found than the other two types.

The normal ridge count of a loop is between 12-14.

On the palm itself it is more usual to find an open-field arrangement of ridges, that is, one where the ridges simply flow with no specific patterning occurring. Complex patterns such as the whorl are less commonly found in the palm.

It is usual to find a mixture of fingerprint patterns in the normal hand.

The normal 'atd' angle is 45 degrees.

The Atypical Hand

In the abnormal hand it is more common to find arches and ulna loops.

On average, there is a lower incidence of ridge count in the atypical hand.

More complex patterns of whorls, loops and composites tend to recur on the palm.

In general, the same pattern occurs on all ten digits.

Because the axial triradius is displaced higher up in the palm, it is often found that the 'atd' angle is greater than 45 degrees.

Apart from mental abnormalities, medical research has linked unusual dermatoglyphic patterns to heart disease, showing a significant correlation between misaligned axial triradii and congenital heart disease. Although the patterns laid down at birth never change, interruptions in the skin ridges themselves may occur through ill-health, dietary deficiency and mental illness. This breaking up of the ridge lines is known as the 'string of pearls' effect (see Figure 28). Interestingly, this 'string of pearls' feature is one factor that seems to crop up amongst schizophrenics. The phenomenon, which does not alter the patterns but merely breaks up the ridging, is symptomatic of ill-health when one's body chemistry is out of sync and the defence mechanism is vulnerable.

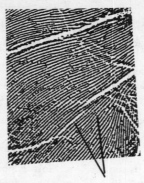

Fig. 28

AIDS is a case in point, where people with the condition have also been found to display the broken ridge effect. On the psychological side, not only people with schizophrenia but also those with milder cases of mental disturbance, such as neurosis, for example, have also been found to possess the same malformed ridging. Recovery or a return to health usually sees the papillary ridges reuniting and restored to form the strong, solid, clear ridge system so characteristic of the healthy hand.

3

The Message in the Lines

The general appearance of the lines in our palms, their condition, construction and composition, give invaluable clues about our mental and physical well-being.

The major lines of **Life**, **Heart** and **Head** are formed during the first few months of foetal development, roughly at the same time as the skin ridge-patterns, or fingerprints, are being stamped in. It is believed by medical researchers that any congenital or chromosomal abnormalities which mark the ridge patterns in characteristic ways may also affect the construction of the main lines at this stage of development as well. Thus, just as fingerprints are genetically handed down from one generation to the next, so the major lines in our hands, too, will be influenced by the DNA package we have inherited from our parents and their parents before them.

But, though formed so early on in our development, contrary to popular myth, our lines can and do change throughout the course of our lives. According to the way we live our lives, to our environmental conditioning, to the decisions we take in life, to our states of health, our lines can grow, increase, change colour, strengthen, weaken, diminish and, in some cases, even disappear altogether. Some changes may take years to come about whilst others, like stress lines across the fingertips for example, can appear and disappear again within a matter of days.

Think of the lines in your hands as channels conducting energy – rather like electric cables in your house. The cables are attached to the mains, pass through the fuse boxes and branch out between walls, floors and ceilings to end in power points on the skirting boards of every room in the house. If this wiring system is in good order and the supply adequate for your requirements, then you know you can confidently plug in whatever appliance you need to use and it will suddenly come to life for you. Flick a switch, and the hi-fi will start blaring out its music; press a button, and the TV will fill the room with moving pictures; turn a knob, and the lights will glow or dim at your command.

But electrical circuits that are not robust enough for the job, cables that are old and cracked or wiring that is faulty in any way means that your hair-dryer or table-lamp are not going to work when you plug them in. In fact, you may well blow a fuse when you overload the system or, worse still, the wiring may spark, start a fire and burn the house down. Worn cables, like lines that are thin, frayed or broken, are a sign of danger and need to be dealt with as soon as possible. Just as the electrician will suck his teeth and shake his head and announce that the whole house has to be rewired, so the hand analyst will advise that action be taken to fortify the lines.

In this way, lines in the hand may be thought of as conductors of energy, as representing your physical wiring system. Good diet, adequate exercise, plenty of rest coupled with a positive attitude to life will keep those channels healthy and in good working order. Stretch your resources, overload the system, abuse your constitution or generally neglect to keep up the running repairs and pretty soon you'll run out of steam; various components such as the liver or the lungs, let's say, may start to show signs of wear and misuse and may eventually pack up altogether.

Signs of such wear and tear, of impending surges of demand upon the system, warnings of possible dangers to come, predisposition to particular ailments or general inherited weak links within our bodies are clearly marked in our hands and easily detectable by the practised eye long before the condition develops into a clinical disease and even well in advance of a stethoscope or blood test picking up signs of trouble.

A fraying line, for example, may warn of the need to shore up our resources, an island may pin-point areas of concern, a bar cutting across a main line will hint at a possible obstruction, whether mental or physical, that is likely to impede the flow of energy and act as a temporary set-back. Bearing in mind that, like the wiring system that takes years to fall into disrepair, diseases don't suddenly happen overnight but take time – sometimes many years – to develop and produce their characteristic symptoms. And because lines can and do change, taking preventive action as soon as we detect their corresponding signs in our hands may mean all the difference between maintaining our good health and succumbing to disease.

But how can you spot the signs early enough? And is intervention always successful?

The first part of the question is easier to answer than the second. But the second part is very much dependent on spotting the signs in the lines early enough, on taking the correct course of action and on the nature of the disease itself.

To begin with, good health is a question of balance and, like the engine in a car, all the components that make up the motor must be synchronized and must function in harmony together, otherwise the timing will be thrown out or one component will start to wear more rapidly than another, producing a domino effect as each part places undue stress on every other in turn.

In just the same way, this idea holds true for your hand because one of the most important underlying principles of hand analysis is that every aspect of a hand must be in good proportion to every other. A mount that is disproportionately large, a finger that is exceptionally short in comparison to the rest, a nail that stands out because it is a different shape, will emphasize the particular characteristic about you that is represented by that feature. An aspect that is discordant, or that jars in any way will, in a sense, throw the whole system out of balance. And this applies in just the same way to your lines as well.

Lines in the palm must suit and match the type of hand in which they are found. If yours do, you will be said to be well-balanced. If they don't, you may experience all sorts of tensions and conflicting emotions. You might find it difficult to take things in your stride, for example. Your reactions to certain situations might be inappropriate or you might give out the wrong signals or cues to other people. In extreme cases there may be what psychologists term 'behavioural problems', with all the aggression and sudden mood swings that go with those conditions where frustrations can build up and give rise to a variety of emotional disorders.

Altogether, it is this very mismatching of the elements in the hand that reflects the internal friction that can undermine your health, both mentally and physically, if the tensions are allowed to go unrecognized and unchecked.

Another important factor in detecting any imbalance that might be occurring in your system is the actual colour of your lines. Too pale or too dark in comparison to the skin of your palm would be symptomatic that all is not well.

But it is the actual construction of your major lines, together with any faults or unexpected markings on them – whether they are thin, brittle, frayed, broken, crossed, islanded, chained or damaged in any way – that will allow us to home in on potential danger spots and raise the alarm. And though not absolutely accurate to the minute, one of the great advantages of hand analysis is that these markings in your lines can be timed by measuring your palm and applying a timing gauge to it. Thus it is that a certain degree of forecasting can be made in just the same way that a doctor might predict the possible onset of disease by noting particular behaviour or specific early-warning symptoms in his or her patients.

For example, current statistics and clinical experience might lead that doctor to warn any of his/her patients who are long-term smokers that if they don't give up smoking their habitual 60 cigarettes a day, there is a strong possibility they will end up with serious lung disease. In just the same way, then, a close examination of future markings in your lines will lead a hand analyst to conclude the *likelihood* of certain outcomes according to your current behaviour, habits and lifestyle, and by using the timing gauge a pretty fair judgement can be made of when your system is *likely* to come under attack, and your health *likely*, if at all, to break down.

But in hand analysis, just as in life, there are pretty few absolutes and it is essential to remember that any markings in your hand simply denote *potential*, *predisposition*, *possibility*. Their mere presence does not imply that a certain event is bound to happen, that any tendency you may show towards a disease is 100 per cent certain to develop into a full-blown clinical or pathological condition. So, just as a doctor may tell his or her patient that, as long as the damage hasn't gone too far, the lungs of the heavy smoker should in time repair themselves, so, too, the hand analyst can tell a client that with a change of behaviour, attitude, lifestyle, etc. there's a very good chance that negative markings can disappear and lines repair themselves as the healing process in the body takes place.

FREE WILL

One of the cardinal rules of hand analysis is that lines can and do change and that we all have free will which we can use to a greater or lesser extent in our lives.

When it comes to health aspects, certain markings in the hands bring to light our susceptibility to illnesses and disease. If, by examining our hands, we discover that we have a tendency towards respiratory problems, let's say, then we may have the power to do something about it if we so wish. By keeping warm, perhaps, by avoiding chills, by not smoking, by seeking prompt medical attention the minute we feel a cold has gone to our chests, we can prevent any bronchial trouble from developing. But if we know we are predisposed to bronchitis and choose to ignore the fact, should we happen to live in a freezing garret, in very damp conditions, chain-smoke and ignore any chest pains that we might feel, then the weakest link, which in this example is the respiratory system, will snap and our lungs will pay the price.

By studying our hands, by measuring and timing the lines, we take control of our own fate, of our own destiny, of our own lives and of our own health. It is by understanding the markings in our hands, by understanding how these relate to the system as a whole and by using our free will that we are enabled to take that control.

A systematic analysis of the lines, then, which will give invaluable clues not only about our predisposition to ill-health, but also show when the likely onset of any problems may be expected, is summarized in the check-list below:

Check-list:
- Full/empty hand
- Matching lines to hand types
- Colour of lines
- Construction of the lines

- Specific markings on the lines
- Timing

FULL HAND vs EMPTY HAND

An instant clue to a person's state of health and, just as importantly, state of mind, lies in what the hand analysts term the 'full' or 'empty' hand. Fullness or emptiness here refers to the quantity of lines that exist in the palm. A full hand, as illustrated in Figure 29a, is unmistakable as it contains a veritable cobweb of lines criss-crossing each other all over palm and fingers, giving the whole hand a rather crowded and confused look. In contrast, the empty hand, as seen in Figure 29b, contains very few lines, often only the three or four major lines, thus giving the palm an uncluttered appearance.

Essentially, the full hand denotes a natural worrier, a highly-strung nature, a person who is hypersensitive, mentally on the go the whole time. Here it is as if the wiring is out of control, as if an excess of electricity is fairly crackling in the atmosphere and far too much energy is scattered about willy-nilly. If you own a full hand you're the sort of person who lives on nervous energy. As a rule of thumb, then, *the more lines in the hand, the more sensitive the individual and the more nervous tension that is generated.*

And it is this heightened sensitivity that makes owners of the full hand so emotional and in direct touch with their nervous systems. They appear to be aware of every little ache and pain, responsive to every change in their physiology, in their circumstances, in their surroundings, in the people with whom they interact. Because the quantity of lines directly correlates with the amount of sensitivity and nervous tension that an individual displays, the more lines that are possessed, the more hypersensitive that individual and the more anxious and fretful the behaviour. The level of neurosis, it could be said, increases proportionately to the number of extraneous lines in the palm. A hand that presents a profuse and complicated pattern of lines, therefore, represents a highly complex personality, someone who is easily suggestible and thus prone to a wide range of psychosomatic disorders.

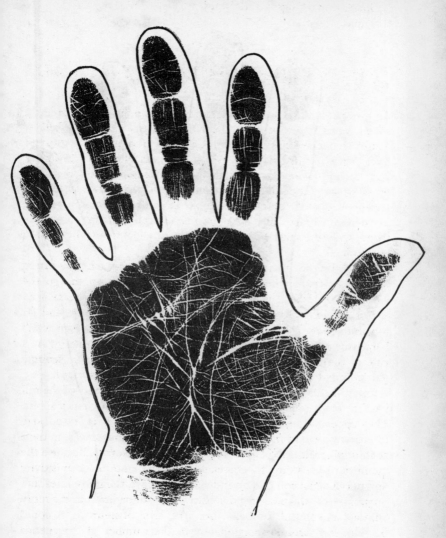

Fig. 29a

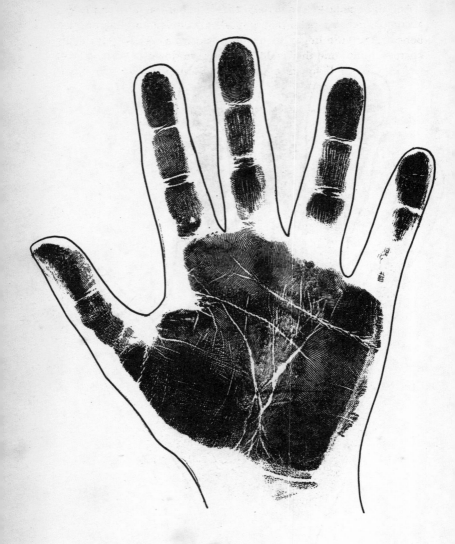

Fig. 29b

And to complicate the matter still further, if the full hand is also accompanied by a palm that is markedly curved and juts out just beneath the little finger, its owner possesses a very fidgety, highly charged mind, one that is difficult to calm down or to switch off (see Figure 30). If you recognize these features in your own hands

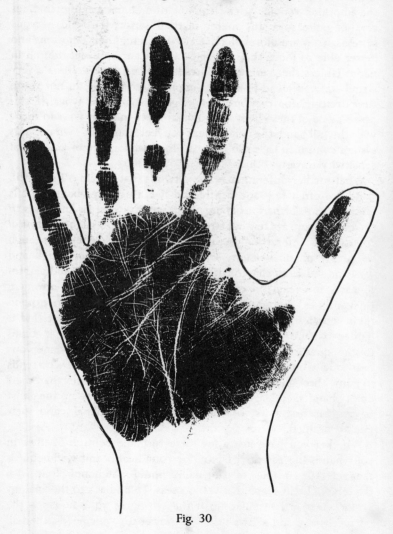

Fig. 30

then yoga, deep-breathing relaxation exercises or some form of meditation will work wonders to help calm your nervous excitement and restore a healthy balance.

In comparison, the fewer and clearer the lines, the more stable is the nervous system and the more balanced the sensitivities and the emotions. People with a clear, uncluttered pattern of main lines are not quite so at the mercy of their sensitivities and nervous systems. They are more effective at controlling their emotions and better able to focus their energies and attention upon the job in hand. Unless there are any contradictory features, such as a very steeply curved Head line for example, these people do not waste time fretting, for they are not in general anxious types. If you possess one of these hands, though stronger in many ways to those with the full hand, the detachment you feel from your own nervous system can mean that you may, at times, lack a certain amount of sensitivity towards others.

What further differentiates these two is that the lines in the full hand are often fine and brittle and it is this very quality that is characteristic of *nervous* energy and activity whereas the lines in the empty hand are few but strong – and strong lines denote *physical* robustness. Interestingly, those with nervous energy, though seemingly physically more fragile, are in fact rather tough and resilient and seem able to withstand difficult situations and painful illnesses for years on end. Conversely, those with the stronger, thicker lines, though physically much stronger, seem to expend their energies in short, sharp bursts and as a consequence find it harder to maintain their strength over a long period. When it comes to the question of health, then, it is often the wiry, nervous individual who is better equipped to withstand pain and who tends to come through a period of ill-health remarkably better than their empty-handed colleagues who may all too readily give up the ghost once their first burst of energy has been discharged and their vitality drained.

Whether you have just a few or a veritable cobweb of lines in your hand, the essential factor for your health and well-being is that the types of lines in your palm should match and blend with the type of hand shape that you possess. Think back to the analogy of the electrical installation: if the wiring in your house is the correct gauge and allows sufficient power for your needs, then all the equipment in your house will run efficiently and well. Should you try, however, to draw too heavily on a system that doesn't have enough capacity to drive all the appliances that you plug in, then you'll simply blow the fuses.

MATCHING LINES TO HAND TYPES

Just as a pair of shoes must suit and, more importantly, must fit you well, so lines in the palm must both suit and fit the type of hand in which they occur. The four categories of hands – **Earth**, **Air**, **Fire** and **Water** – are each associated with particular types of lines and each with a particular quality and formation of lines. Like a well-made and well-fitting pair of shoes, where the lines suit the hand type an easy relationship will co-exist between mind, body and spirit. But, like an ill-fitting pair of shoes which pinch and chafe the feet, where the lines mismatch, that relationship may not be quite so comfortable.

For example, too many fine and wispy lines in an Earth hand would be as ill-matched as too few very strong lines in a Water hand. Both would present a complex situation where the wiring and energy demands would be at variance with the needs of their owners. Using the shoe analogy again, a jumble of wispy lines in the Earth hand would be like trying to keep on a pair of shoes that were three sizes too big. The consequences of this is not hard to imagine – distorting toes in an attempt to keep the things on, blisters from rubbing as the shoes slip, constantly tripping over yourself and losing your balance.

Similarly, few but boldly engraved lines in the Water hand have their parallel in shoes that are too small and too tight. Here the toes become distorted as they are cramped into too narrow a space, and the whole foot and ankle are in danger of swelling up as the blood-flow becomes constricted. And so it is that, just as every part of the hand must be in proportion to every other, it is equally essential that the lines, too, must be in harmonious agreement with the environment in which they are found.

The **EARTH** hand, representing as it does a solid, down-to-earth, practical, hard-working individual, is characteristically accompanied by few lines, although these stand out in the palm because they are usually boldly marked and firmly etched (see Figure 31).

- If this hand contains very few lines which are remarkably strong and thick, the individual will display physical strength but unless he or she is able to channel it properly that power may run out of control. Such people are able to put on great spurts of energy which then rapidly burn themselves out, leaving their owners depleted and exhausted.
- Weak, broken lines in this type of hand would rob its owner of a great deal of physical robustness, so whilst she wants to work from dawn to dusk, she would lack the energies and the recuperative abilities that her fundamental nature demands of her.
- Similarly, a cobweb effect of fine lines in this palm would reflect a great deal of sensitivity and a highly-strung nature at variance with the Earth hand's basic common-sense and pragmatic view of life. People possessing the Earth hand shape could be described as externalizers, they are very up-front. Their thought processes, their emotions, their interactions with others, with situations and with their environment are all conducted 'externally'. With the average Earth type, what-you-see-is-what-you-get. There are no deep hidden recesses, if you like. Lots of lines in this hand, though, would denote a tendency to internalize which is so alien to the fundamental nature of this group. So, whilst this would make the Earth individual more sensitive than the norm, it is this very sensitivity that would give rise to a good deal of inner tension.
- Though the Earth hand category is usually associated with the manual worker, when the hand does contain a good many lines it denotes a mentality able to blend intellectual and creative thought, one where its owner is not only able to think imaginatively but also to put those ideas into reality.

The **AIR** hand represents a breezy, lively and buzzing personality for whom variety is the spice of life. Communications and

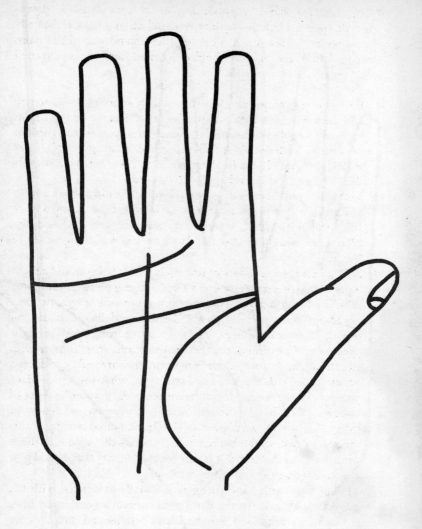

Fig. 31
THE EARTH HAND

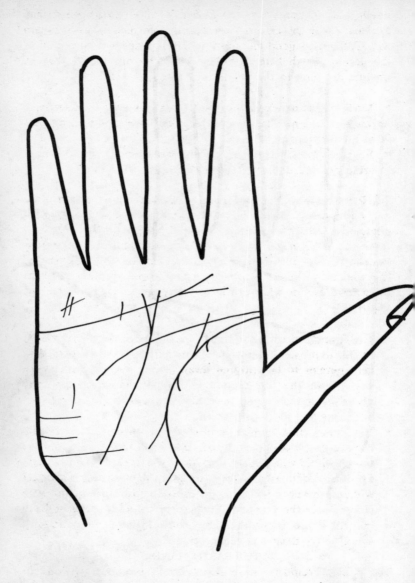

Fig. 32
THE AIR HAND

intellectual pursuits are preferred in life. Characteristically associated with this category are clear, well-formed lines (see Figure 32). Certainly, a good few more would be expected here than in the average Earth hand but they would be distinct, leaving an uncluttered look to the palm.

- Too few lines here would suggest a lack of sensitivity. Creativity, intellectual appreciation and the gift of invention would suffer as a consequence.
- Too many lines, particularly if badly constructed, would perhaps bring out the neurotic in this character.

The **FIRE** hand typifies a live wire, exuberant, outgoing, optimistic and enthusiastic. People possessing this hand expend masses of energy, for they throw themselves heart and soul into whatever it is they are doing at the time. Typically, the Fire hand possesses many lines and though the main ones will in general be strongly engraved they may, nevertheless, be interwoven by several minor ones which often have a somewhat brittle and fragmented appearance (see Figure 33).

- The stronger the lines in this hand, the more the owner would be able to muster her powers of concentration rather than allow her energies to be frittered away. Strong, well-cut lines here would give the Fire-handed individual enough mental and physical resources together with plenty of scope to bring his or her plans and ideas to fruition.
- Too many fine lines, particularly if broken and poorly constructed, would perhaps be considered rather dangerous to this character who already lives life in the fast lane anyway. Such a profusion of lines would suggest a very highly-strung individual with too much sensitivity, too much impulsiveness, too little control over the emotions. Judgement would be poor and the individual too impressionable. Physical fuses, quite literally, would be in danger of blowing.

The **WATER** hand is unmistakable for its profusion of lines. In general the main ones are finely formed and criss-crossed with a great many extraneous lines which are often thin, brittle and

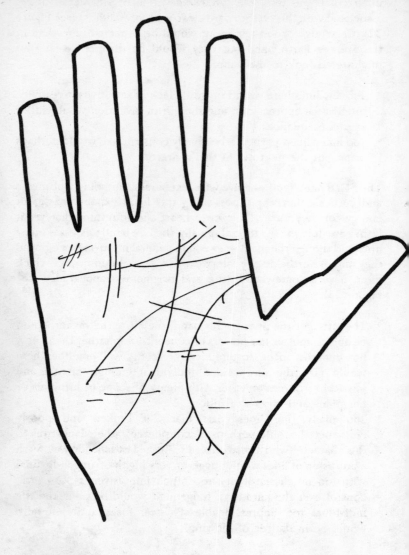

Fig. 33
THE FIRE HAND

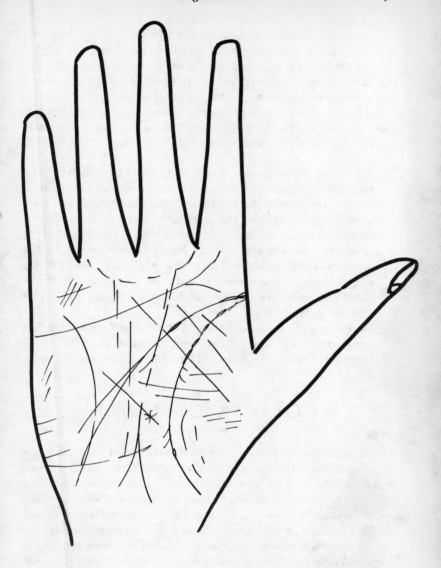

Fig. 34
THE WATER HAND

fragmented (see Figure 34). Hypersensitivity is the main characteristic of those possessing this type of hand for they are people who live very close to their emotions and are highly responsive to the moods and feelings of others. As opposed to the Earth hand types, these people are internalizers: they experience the world very much from within. To say they are complex doesn't even come half-way towards describing their inner selves. Indeed, these people have hidden depths, labyrinthine passages too tortuous and complicated for some – even they themselves – to fathom.

- The more lines in this hand, the more highly-strung the individual. Depression and all manner of mental instability is likely to affect the owners of these hands. Such people are likely to fret and worry over the least trifle and as a consequence display the sort of behaviour that might be described as obsessional or neurotic. Though highly creative as a rule, too many lines in this hand will show that whilst talent is plentiful, attention and concentration is scattered. Consequently, clever plans may never see the light of day and brilliant ideas never brought to fruition.
- In the unlikely event of finding a Water hand containing few lines, there will be greater determination to fulfill one's ambitions, though a certain cold-blooded ruthlessness may exist.

COLOUR OF LINES

The colour of your lines should be slightly darker than your skin but should generally match in tone. European hands ideally contain dark pink lines; black and Asian hands are graced with browny-beige lines set in pinkish-beige palms. However, care must be taken when making judgements about the colour of lines for not only should the race of the owner be taken into account, but also the ambient temperature and, just as importantly, whatever activity has preceeded the analysis. If you've been energetically working out in a gym, for example, you might expect that your lines, and the colour of your whole hand in general, will be a good deal pinkier than if you'd been defrosting your chest freezer for the past couple of hours! So please do use your common sense when you're making this assessment.

- When the lines are very red, regardless of race or activity, it is a sign not only of a fiery temperament but, in terms of health, of feverish conditions or cardio-vascular problems.
- Yellowy lines in a European hand may suggest liver problems and jaundice in particular.
- Lines that appear pale or run white when the fingers are flexed back and the skin across the palm stretched, may well signify a deficiency of iron. Many women find that their lines tend to lose colour during, and a few days following, menstruation. This is directly a result of iron loss. An increased intake of iron alone may not in some cases be sufficient to redress the balance. When the white lines persist it may be that magnesium and Vitamin B6 are also deficient. Vitamins belonging to the B-complex, C and E may help to restore the balance. Folic acid, too, often given in conjunction with iron tablets to pregnant women, helps the absorption and assimilation of this essential mineral.
- Generally speaking, pale lines mean that vitality and physical resources are low. Rest and an improved diet containing a good balance of vitamins and minerals should be enough to restore the lines to their normal colour.
- Sometimes, in certain terminal diseases, the lines may fade away. This condition has also been found to occur in cases where there is a severe copper deficiency. However, given the Western diet, it is unlikely that this condition will be found in the more developed nations of the world.
- Lines have also been found to disappear in rare cases where physical damage has occurred to the brain, but have reappeared again once health is restored. Yet the hands of mummified bodies, dead for some thousands of years, have been found quite remarkably still to show signs of their major lines. As an example, Figure 35 is a print of a female hand taken six days after death. Note that her lines are still showing clearly.

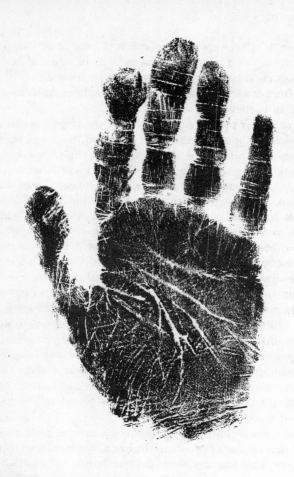

Fig. 35

RIGHT- AND
LEFT-HANDEDNESS

Many people are confused about right- and left-handedness – and no wonder when silly myths and old wives' tales on the subject abound! 'The left is what you're born with and the right is what you make of yourself' is the typical sort of thing you might hear time and again. And the fact that the word 'left' in Latin implies *sinister malevolence* has meant that for centuries left-handers have been considered evil, untrustworthy, villainous people – something which, as you can imagine, hasn't helped their image one little bit.

Fortunately, psychologists working in this very area have done a sterling job in clearing up the whole issue of right- and left-handedness and, in the process, have completely vindicated the poor, long-suffering left-hander.

In brief, what the research has found is that roughly between 12 and 13 per cent of people in the Western world are left-handed, and of those slightly more tend to be male than female. More importantly, tests have shown that the two hemispheres of our brain control very different functions. The left side deals with what might loosely be termed 'hard core' subjects such as the logical and rational processes that we require in order to read, write and calculate. The right hemisphere meanwhile deals with the 'softer' processes, with our intuitive and emotional responses, our ability creatively to appreciate our environment, art, music and suchlike.

Now, what is fascinating is that commands from these two sides of our brain cross over and control the opposite side of our bodies, so that our left hemisphere controls our right eye, ear, arm, hand, leg, foot and so on through the right side of the body whilst the right brain hemisphere controls our left side. And this is why the majority of us write with our right hands, see better with our right eyes, kick a football with our right foot, etc. Our right hand, then, becomes known as our dominant or active hand, whereas the left is our passive hand.

When it comes to left-handers, the difference is that the roles of their two hemispheres are simply reversed. It is their right hemisphere that deals with the 'hard core' subjects and that controls their left sides. And so it is that their left hands become their dominant ones. Simple as that. Nothing more sinister or demoniacal - just a geographical reversal of roles in the brain.

These findings not only do an excellent PR job for left-handers but they also help to clarify the picture for hand analysts and confirm what we have known all along about the differences between the two hands. Firstly, each hand contains specific information - the passive (controlled by the 'intuitive', 'emotional' hemisphere) tells about such things as our instinctive reactions, our potential, our private selves, or what might be called our *anima*. The active or dominant hand (controlled by the 'logical', 'rational' hemisphere) tells us about our public selves, our *persona*, whether we have developed our potential or not, as the case may be. So, not only do we recognize that information may differ between one hand and the other, we are also aware that sometimes the information may even conflict.

Why it is so important to understand the differences between our two hands is because when it comes to analysing the markings that specifically concern health matters, we must clearly differentiate between the two findings. The markings in our passive hands will tell us about our inherited predispositions to disease, our weak links, if you like. These show what could happen if we were sorely to abuse our systems. The markings in our active or dominant hands show the sort of illnesses that are more likely to develop.

But the two hands must be taken together because there could just as well be positive markings in the passive hand which could offset any negative information found in the active one. When both hands show the same adverse marking on the same corresponding spot, that is when the odds would seem more stacked in favour of the illness or breakdown in health taking place.

But even then, we cannot be 100 per cent sure that the event will come about because we must remember that lines do change. And to squash yet another old wives' tale, the lines change on *both* hands - left as well as right - although the passive hand does tend to change more slowly.

CONSTRUCTION OF
THE LINES

Ideally, the best type of line, be it Life, Head, Heart, Apollo or whatever, should be clearly etched, not too thick nor too thin, and free from any sort of obstruction or impediment such as islands or cross-bars.

- Thick and deeply chiselled lines show robust physical vitality, plenty of power and energy. However, this type of line suggests a lack of control over one's strength and though the vitality is plentiful in short bursts, there is a tendency for the power to burn itself out quickly and so its owner is unable to sustain impetus and momentum at the same level over a long period of time. Such individuals need to learn to pace themselves, not to throw all their reserves into whatever problem is immediately before them, but to modify and temper their energies in a slow burn otherwise they will simply deplete their resources and end up completely exhausted.

- Very thin, fine lines show a brittle vitality and, like a thin electric cable, suggest an inability to support great surges of energy when required. Owners of such lines may not have a lot of physical or mental resources at their disposal, so that if extra demands were to be made upon them, such as might occur during a time of emotional crisis, let's say, these people might very well buckle under the strain.

- Lines that are fuzzy or woolly in appearance show a lack of concentration (see Figure 36). People with this type of line are unable to focus their energies constructively but tend to scatter their abilities and their strengths.

MARKINGS ON THE LINES

Any fault or marking in the line, whether it is an island, crossbar or whatever, will represent an obstacle to the normal smooth

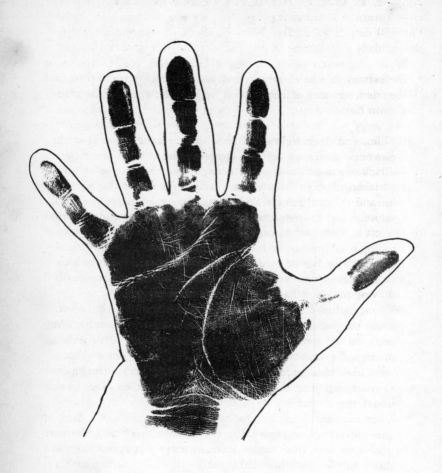

Fig. 36

running of the energies denoted by that line. So an island in your Life line, for example, will suggest a period when your physical constitution is running at a low ebb, whereas one in your Head line will denote an undercurrent of stress, of worry and anxiety that is likely to continue throughout the duration of that marking.

- **Crossbars** as a rule represent opposition or obstruction from outside forces (see *a* in Figure 37). A short crossing bar that cuts a main line acts rather like a dam in a river and stops the flow of energy. The strength, length and thickness of the crossbar is significant in denoting the sort of impact the event will have on its owner. The longer and stronger one will obviously rock the individual a good deal more than one that is short and fine. Invariably, however, this marking is indicative of a temporary set-back and the condition of the line after the crossbar needs to be closely examined in order to determine whether the obstruction has left any long-term damage or not. If, immediately after the crossing bar, the main line picks up with the same strength and vigour as before, then the individual should recover fairly quickly from any adverse effects represented by that marking. But if, directly following the marking, the main line should break, fray or form itself into an island, then the chances are that the set-back will have much greater consequences and will be more likely to take its toll on the owner's health. The nature of the obstruction represented by the crossbar and its effect on the individual can be determined firstly by which main line it appears in, secondly by its strength, and thirdly by examining the other main lines to see if any adverse markings appear on those as well at around the same time.

- A tiny cluster of crossbars (see *b* in Figure 37) that cut the line at the same spot so that they form a **star-burst** effect suggest a shock to the system, and the nature of that shock, whether physical or psychological, very much depends on the line in which they occur. Consider this formation as a fuse that blows – but only when the pattern occurs *on a line*. In some hands stars may be found free-standing on the mounts quite independent of any of the lines, and in general these are positive markings, more concerned with character and disposition rather than giving information which might have a direct bearing on health.

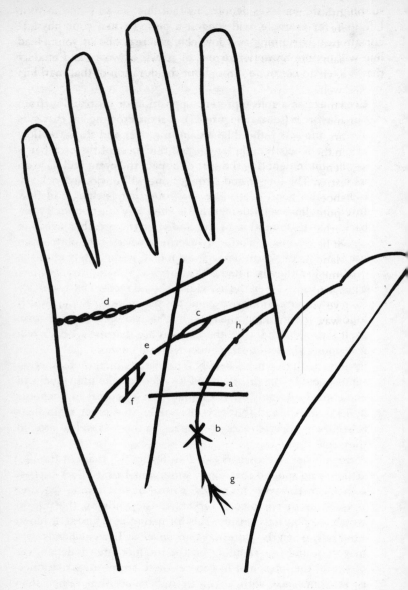

Fig. 37

- **Islands** in the line denote a lowering of energy levels (see *c* in Figure 37). Here it is as if the channel of power has been split into two, each branch halving the force and thus detracting from its main impetus and thrust. Throughout the duration of an island, then, vitality and resistances are low and the individual's health and well-being become susceptible to attack. This impaired energy level might affect its owner's mental performance, physical health or emotional well-being, according to the line in which the island occurs. By measuring and timing the line it is possible to calculate when the lowered resistance is likely to occur and, by measuring the length of the island itself, how long the condition is likely to last. When an island in one of your lines is detected well in advance, it is worthwhile planning a strategic campaign to offset any potentially adverse effects that might occur in the future. So perhaps taking up yoga or some form of meditation, let's say, might help you to prevent serious stress from building up should an island be spotted in your Head line. Equally, one in your Life line might call for a review of your diet, perhaps, or a radical change to your way of life, or urge you perhaps to ask your doctor to give you a general check-up. By using advance strategies in this way, it is possible to dodge any problems that might arise in the future. As a result, you may even find that your island will disappear altogether.

- A **chain** in a line is basically a series of islands and shows poor vitality (see *d* in Figure 37). Chained formations within the major lines may often be a sign of mineral deficiencies.

- **Breaks** in the line show change (see *e* in Figure 37). Essentially, a broken line denotes the end of one phase in the person's life and the beginning of another. Examining the strength and direction of the new section of line after the break will reveal whether the new phase continues with the same gusto as before, whether there is likely to be greater improvement of circumstances, or whether indeed the subject will begin to experience restrictions in her life. Though usually a break is interpreted as a personal or psychological change in the affairs and circumstances of the individual, there are certain cases, however, such as a break in the Heart line or a particular type of break in a Life line, where this marking can alert its owner to the possibility of a serious health problem.

- Four little lines that form themselves into a **square** formation, either sitting directly over the line or adjoining it by one of its sides, is often a sign of protection (see *f* in Figure 37). Should the square occur over a break or a star formation, for example, it denotes that some form of good fortune or preservation will be at work to mitigate against any very adverse effects that may be represented by those markings. If you find a square attached to one of your lines, you're likely to find that life is rather tough-going throughout the duration of that marking because of an increased work-load and also because the square may be interpreted symbolically as a box, or even as a cell, which suggests a feeling of constriction whilst the formation is in place. However, not all is bleak because another aspect of this marking is that there will be compensations to lighten the load. Timing the line on which the square occurs will show the onset and duration of this period.

- **Fraying** or **tasselling** can appear towards the end of a main line and looks as if the line is feathered (see *g* in Figure 37). When this feature occurs it denotes a scattering, a frittering away of energies. Obviously, then, vitality will be low during this time as the physical and mental power is not being harnessed or channelled properly. If this is seen in your hand it is a warning not to overdo things but rather to consolidate your strengths until your normal levels of energy are restored.

- **Spots, dots** or tiny **indentations**, rather like pin-pricks in the line, show a concentrated period of inner tension or mental stress (see *h* in Figure 37). How this will actually affect the health will vary according to whichever of your lines the marking is in.

LINES AND TIMES

Timing dates and events on the lines can be a tricky business because hands come in all shapes and sizes. As you can imagine, then, it isn't possible to simply apply the same scale to each person because someone with a long palm would register 150 years on her Fate line, say, in comparison to a short-palmed Fate line which would only stretch to a bare 40.

In order to take size into account, then, the scale has to be customized for each individual hand, compressing it to fit a small palm and stretching it out to accommodate a longer one.

Obviously, this aspect of analysing a hand can be difficult at first and this is where experience does pay off, but there are, nevertheless, a few tricks or 'rules of thumb' (explained below) which should help the beginner.

But whether you are just starting out or have been analysing hands for many years, there is a fail-safe system which all the experts not only recommend, but use themselves. Look for a big event marking registering something that happened in the subject's past, time it using the timing gauge and then simply ask the individual to confirm it. If you're a year or two out, adjust the scale to fit and reapply it to another major marker. It really doesn't take very long to get one's eye in and after only a comparatively short time a pretty good level of accuracy can be reached.

The ability to time potential future events accurately has obvious benefits especially when considering aspects of health. One of the principal advantages, of course, is that it is possible to tell when someone's resistances to disease are low and counsel that individual to take care at that time. Another is that you can spot when the onset of a problem is likely to occur so that with advance warning preventive steps can be taken. Forewarned is forearmed!

Not all the lines are suitable for timing, though. The Heart line, for example, is not reliable for this measure nor indeed are any of the other secondary lines, so in general these tend to be avoided. The best results, however, can be obtained by measuring the major lines of Life, Head and Fate and any developments or markings on these lines can be picked out with an impressively good degree of precision.

Though it is possible to measure the lines in the living hand and make quick mental calculations whilst an individual has his or her hand spread out in front of you, it is perhaps more advisable to take a print and to work from that. Instructions on taking clear handprints may be found in the Appendix.

- Figure 38 illustrates how to time events on the **Life line**. A vertical line is drawn from the inside edge of the index finger and extended downwards until it reaches the Life line. This point

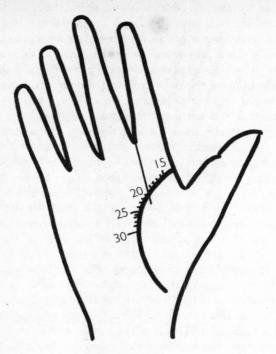

Fig. 38

is roughly 20 years of age. One year of life is represented on the line by about one millimetre – although this very much depends on whether the hand is large or small. If it is large then perhaps the millimetre should be a generous one, whilst if working with a smaller hand the measurement should be compressed a little to slightly less than a millimetre. So the general rule is that a millimetre, more or less, is the unit of measurement that accounts for roughly twelve months. Working from the 20-year mark on the line, one millimetre before that takes us to 19, one more to 18, and so on, backwards towards the edge of the palm. Working forwards from the 20-year mark and down towards the wrist, every millimetre adds on one more year.

• The **Head line** is divided up in the same way, as illustrated in Figure 39. The vertical line is again dropped from the inside edge

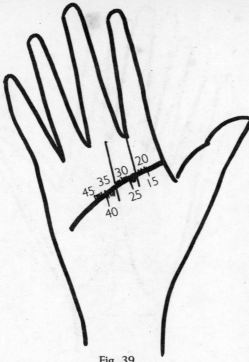

Fig. 39

of the index finger to strike the Head line at 20. The same rule of one-millimetre-to-a-year is applied working backwards from the 20-year mark towards the thumb edge and forwards across the palm from 20 onwards. An additional check that the system is working correctly can be made by dropping a vertical line from the centre of the middle finger down onto the Head line, and this point should touch at around 35 years.

- The **Fate line** is treated somewhat differently. Here, the actual palm itself is measured and then the measurements are transferred across to the line. It is slightly more complicated than timing the other two main lines principally because the Fate line has such a variety of starting points. In some hands it begins attached to the Life line, in others it takes root from the Luna mount. Sometimes it rises almost from the wrist whilst in other

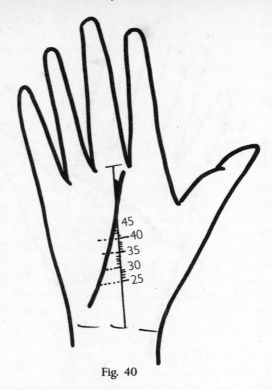

Fig. 40

hands it doesn't appear until well past the Head line. So, with such a diversity of starting points, it is necessary to measure the palm, which at least is a constant, and then to match the Fate line itself onto that scale. Here, the palm is measured by drawing a vertical line from the top rascette, or bracelet, at the wrist to the point where it joins the base of the middle finger. Half-way up is the 35-year-point and a mark should be made on the line to denote the spot. Again, using the millimetre-a-year rule the line is divided off from the wrist up to the 35-year mark. Now here a little poetic licence has to be used because each millimetre is a generous one between 0 to 35, but the scale has to be compressed from 35 up so that each year from the mid-point onwards is represented by a fraction less than one whole millimetre. Once the years have been marked off on the vertical line they can be transferred across by drawing a horizontal line from any given point along the vertical line to strike the Fate line. Figure 40 illustrates how the timing gauge is adapted and applied to this line.

PATTERNS OF HEALTH IN THE MAJOR LINES

The major lines are known as the Life, Heart and Head and studies show that they are formed in that order around the fourth month of foetal development. In some cases, the Fate line, which is also considered a major line, may be formed later on in the developmental process although many new-born babies are still without the line, being found to develop it some years after birth. However, there are just as many babies who are born already possessing a complete set of major lines, together with a full complement of minor ones as well. Figure 41 illustrates these four lines.

Of the minor lines, the one that will tell us a great deal about our health has to be the Hepatica, also known as the Liver line but perhaps best recognized as the Health line. However, it cannot be stressed enough that *all* lines are important and have a role to play, each making its contribution, no matter how big or how small, to the whole pattern of our health and well-being. So ancillary lines, like the Girdle of Venus or the Via Lascivia, act as individual pieces of the jigsaw which must be interpreted in order to see a clearer picture of the whole. Figure 42 illustrates the minor lines in the hand.

LINE CHARACTERISTICS
Comparing the strength of the major lines in our hands is always an interesting exercise and yields fruitful information about our reserves of energy and in which area of our lives we tend to deploy those energies most. In some people's hands the main lines are equally balanced but in many others it is quite remarkable how one line tends to stand out amongst the rest, either because it is

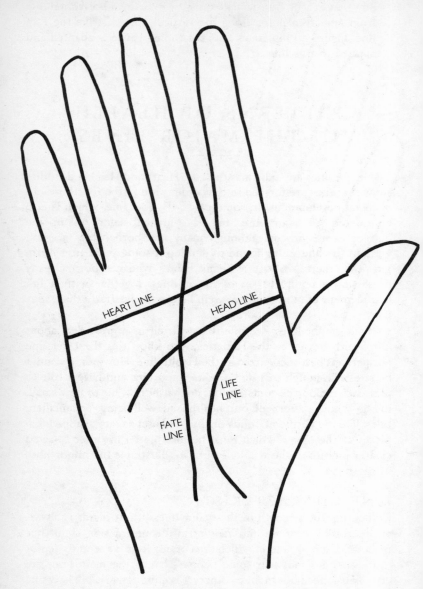

HEART LINE

HEAD LINE

LIFE LINE

FATE LINE

Fig. 41

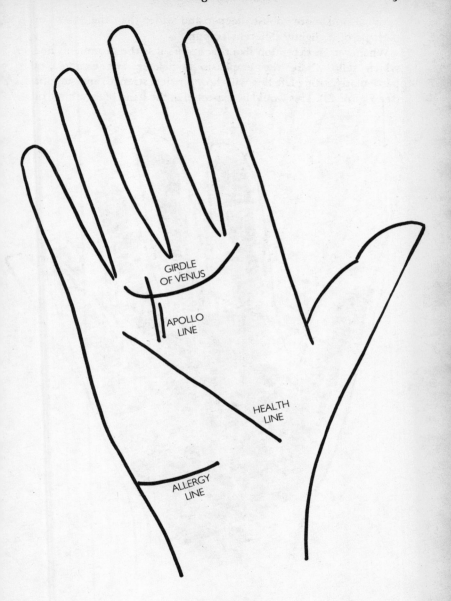

GIRDLE
OF VENUS

APOLLO
LINE

HEALTH
LINE

ALLERGY
LINE

Fig. 42

stronger and more robust, deeper and wider than the others or perhaps of a slightly different colour.

Whenever an exception like this occurs it is the prominent line which tells where the emphasis is placed. For example, a particularly strong Life line will show physical strength and stamina (see Figure 43). This would be expected in the hand of an athlete or

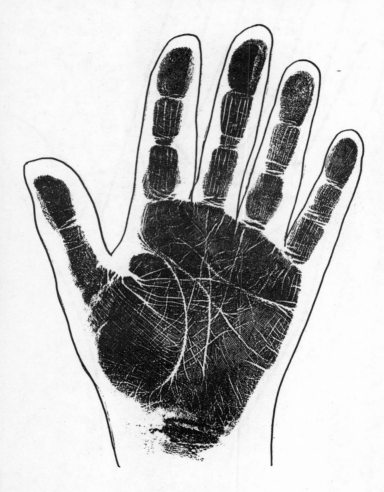

Fig. 43

similarly sporty individual. A prominent Life line tells of masses of physical reserves, there to be tapped whenever the owner requires.

If the Head line is the strongest, as in Figure 44, the mental energies are the driving force of that individual. Mental activity characterizes those possessing a prominent Head line – perhaps

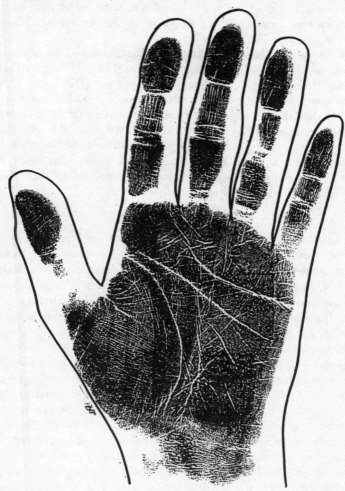

Fig. 44

they're people who do a great deal of thinking, of intellectual work, people whose minds tend to be constantly on the go. What these individuals have to bear in mind is not to let their busy minds push their bodies further than they can go. If their hands show that their physical stamina cannot keep pace with their mental drive they may well overtax their systems and simply end up completely exhausting themselves. Plenty of rest and relaxation in order to let your body catch up, then, is essential if your Head line noticeably stands out in your hand.

As far as the Heart line is concerned, where this line is disproportionately emphasized in the palm, it would suggest that its owner tends to let her heart rule her head (see Figure 45). Excitement, impetuosity and enthusiasm are characteristic of those bearing this feature, and it is this very impulsiveness, this throwing themselves so totally, heart and soul, into whatever they do that can lead not only to mental and physical exhaustion but also to accidents and injuries too. Mistakes, bad judgements and all manner of emotional and psychological complications can also arise due to such impulsive tendencies.

THE LIFE LINE

The Life line denotes the quality or tenor of our lives. This line records both our genetic inheritance and our *awareness* of our physical strength and general state of health. Anything that is likely to sap our strength, to interfere with our progress and development, to affect us physically, emotionally or psychologically in such a way that our health comes under attack, will be registered here in this line by specific negative markings.

Contrary to old wives' tales, the Life line does not indicate longevity; instead, what is important here is the actual construction and composition of the line, as this represents our physical resources. In short, the strength of our Life line is equal to the strength of our constitution and it is this which represents the amount of stamina and vitality that we possess. A poorly formed Life line, with chains, islands and crossbars intercepting it throughout, will describe someone whose vitality is low and thus prone to all sorts of diseases and ill-health. A strong and healthy Life line represents the essential springboard from which all other activity in life can take place.

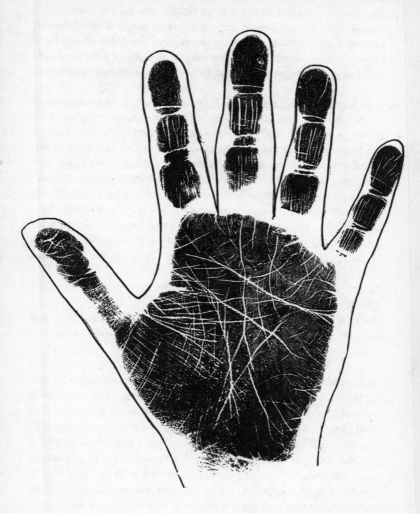

Fig. 45

Location: The Life line is the semi-circular line that sweeps around the thumb. In some hands it hugs tightly around the base of the thumb whilst in others it makes a broad arc out towards the centre of the palm. It begins on the edge of the palm somewhere between the thumb and index finger and proceeds down the hand and around to end at the base of the palm near the wrist.

Psychological indications: A Life line that is widely separated from the Head line at its beginning (as illustrated in Figure 46a) shows a reckless and impulsive nature and thus one with a tendency to accidents and injuries. But one that is joined to the Head line for a considerable distance denotes sensitivity and reticence (see Figure 46b). With this formation a certain shyness or a marked lack of self-confidence resulting in a withdrawn personality can remain with that individual right through into adulthood, interfering with his emotional development, frustrating his intellectual potential and sometimes even blighting his chances of leading a truly independent life. Quite a different matter is the Life line which begins on the Mars mount, close to the base of the thumb (see Figure 46c) and which then arches upwards before regaining its sweep around the ball of the thumb – for in this case hot-headedness and temper tantrums might be the response to expect from its owner.

Physiological indications: The strength of the line corresponds to the strength of our physical constitution. A strong, well-constructed Life line denotes robust health, good vitality, plenty of vigour and physical energy. When weak and poorly formed, interrrupted by islands and breaks, suspect poor vitality and a general lack of zest which manifests itself in a weakened constitution and a susceptibility to poor health. A line that is uneven (as in Figure 47) throughout its length, sometimes appearing strong and deep whilst at other times thin and weak, will denote patchy health, periods when the individual feels strong and robust followed by times when energy is low and resistance to disease is poor. If you possess this type of see-sawing effect it is a warning that you tend to take on too much during the 'strong' periods, overtaxing your resources thus depleting

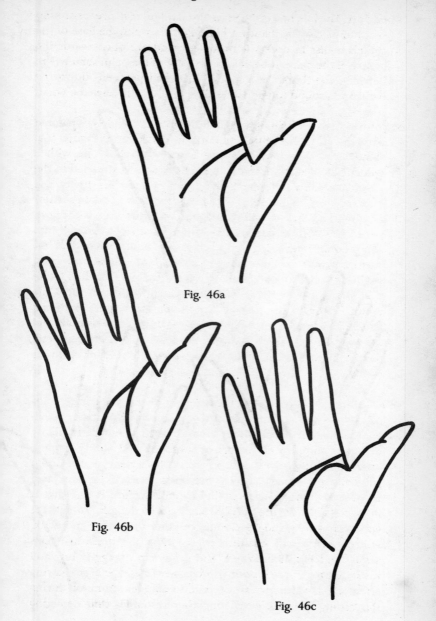

Fig. 46a

Fig. 46b

Fig. 46c

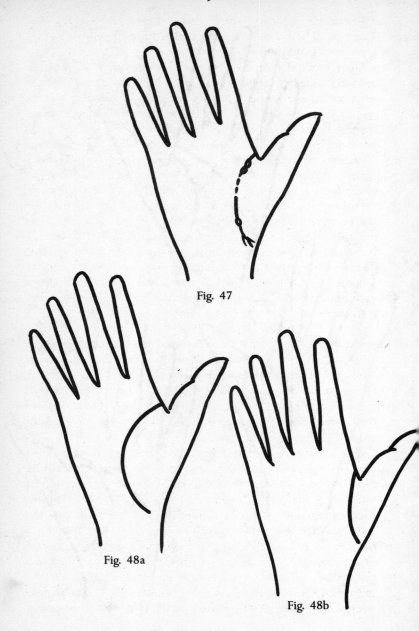

Fig. 47

Fig. 48a

Fig. 48b

your energies, as denoted by the 'weakened' sections of the line. This type of line is warning you to pace yourself better and find a proper equilibrium within your routine.

Apart from the construction of the line itself, its journey around the ball of the thumb will reveal the amount of physical resources at our disposal. A wide sweep where the line arcs its way to the centre of the palm means that it encircles a large expanse of the area known as the mount of Venus (see Figure 48a). Because this area represents the energy store, such a formation would indicate plenty of reserves, good resistance against disease and excellent powers of recuperation. Conversely, a line that closely follows the root of the thumb means that the mount of Venus will be thin and meagre and thus the energy store will not be great (see Figure 48b). Such an indication, then, would imply low energy levels, a lack of resistance to disease, poor recuperative powers and general delicacy of health. A narrow Life line such as this also suggests a limited sex drive and there is also a hint here of difficulties with conception and, in extreme cases, possible frigidity and impotence.

Length: Much worry has centred around the question of length of the Life line, particularly since a short line has been mistakenly reputed to indicate a short life. The length of our Life lines *do not* correspond to the length of our lives. Indeed, many elderly people have been found to possess short Life lines whilst many with long lines have died long before those lines showed any signs of terminating.

Very few true short Life lines exist because more often than not, when examined closely, an apparently short line will be found to be connected by a fine hairline to a new section of Life line, either further out towards the centre of the palm or overlapping another on the inside, situated closer towards the thumb. What this in fact constitutes is not a short line but a break in the line, and a broken line essentially represents a break of continuity. Psychologically, a broken Life line will denote a change of direction, a change of circumstances within the individual's life. Physiologically, a break here might well denote a serious health problem, possibly an injury or a life-threatening disease. This feature, together with its implications and markings that might reveal mitigating circumstances, is discussed in more detail below.

It is probably just as well to be reminded at this point that lines can and do change and this means they can grow as well. Indeed, some children do possess short Life lines as babies which then grow in length as the child herself matures and develops. And not only do they lengthen with age but they can also strengthen up and consolidate, too. Many handprints taken at regular intervals from childhood to adult will show that early weak, islanded lines can mature in time into lines that are solid, healthy and robust.

SPECIFIC MARKINGS IN THE LINE

Any markings relating to health in the Life line can be timed with a good degree of accuracy so that, if detected early enough, preventive action may be taken, early diagnosis sought if necessary and the health generally bolstered so as to resist or avoid altogether the stresses and strains that can so adversely affect the system.

Markings are usually very clearly stamped but when analysing their significance it is essential, firstly, to compare and contrast all the other major lines at the same corresponding point in time, and secondly, to check the appearance of the line immediately following the marking. If the line is strong and clear after the marking, there is unlikely to be any lasting detrimental effect. If, however, the other main lines show similar indications, and the Life line is weakened or impaired after the marking, the message is clearly one that steps should be taken to try to avert the situation. Quite often a change of attitude, modifications to the diet or changes in the way of life have been known to make dramatic alterations to the lines in the hand and, with such positive action, negative markings have disappeared and the main lines restored to health.

- **Islands**, which are frequently found in the Life line, denote a weakening of the constitution - energy levels lowered and resistance down. Depending on its position in the line, an island can point to specific areas of concern and may either indicate a temporary state of affairs, lasting only for the duration of the island itself, or may represent a general predisposition to a particular disease.

Many Life lines are joined at their beginning with the Head line and in some hands, where these two intertwine, they form a series of little islands, or a chain effect (see *a* in Figure 49). This early section of the line represents our childhood and early years of life and either of two interpretations have been found to apply to islands occurring here. The first interpretation suggests that the island denotes a period of worry and anxiety, a troubled childhood, perhaps – problems with parents, unhappiness at school, undue pressures, uncertainty over future directions in life. Any of these can appear insurmountable problems when we're young and our minds still impressionable, and the implications that are represented by the islands may well have repercussions elsewhere in the hand and even echo through into our adult lives.

The second interpretation that can be applied is to do with physical health and implies that those possessing the island in this position succumb to more than their fair share of childhood illnesses. Moreover, this formation suggests a general predisposition to bronchial and respiratory problems so that if you possess islands at the beginning of your Life line you will be more susceptible than others to chest infections and illnesses such as asthma, bronchitis, sinusitis, allergies affecting the respiratory tract and all manner of ailments connected with the lungs.

Occurring lower down the line (see *b* in Figure 49), an island here is associated with back and spinal problems. If you are one of the many who suffer with backache there may well be an island present in this part of your Life line in your hand.

Lower down still (see *c* in Figure 49), an island in the Life line may represent general debility, a state where the health is run down and therefore becomes vulnerable to many of the diseases that affect the middle-aged. Urological or gynaecological problems may be depicted in this way, as well as illnesses affecting the alimentary canal, the cardio-vascular system and a whole host of other organic problems that seem to manifest themselves at that time of life.

Speculation exists that a tiny, well-formed, oval-shaped island

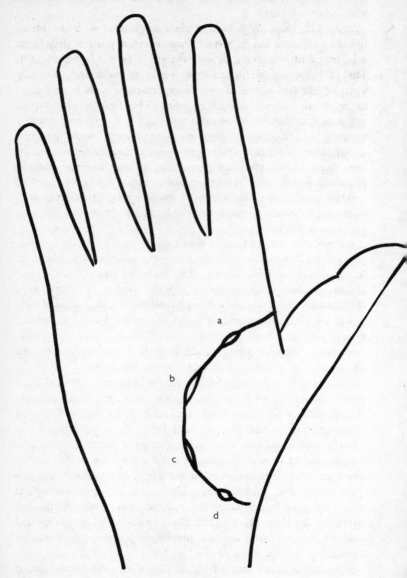

Fig. 49

found on the Life line at the base of the palm near the wrist (see *d* in Figure 49) may imply a predisposition to cancer. This theory, however, is a long way from being proven and requires a great deal more research before we can confirm its significance. Remembering, firstly, that an island reflects a splitting of our energy which weakens our constitution and allows us to become vulnerable to disease, secondly, that an island situated so far along the line represents old age, and thirdly, that by and large cancer is a disease somewhat more prevalent amongst the elderly, it can be seen how such a marking could conceivably be correlated with cancer. However, until more research is properly carried out and more corroborating evidence is collected, this theory must be treated as purely speculative at this stage.

What must always be borne in mind is the fact that with a careful diet, plenty of rest, appropriate exercise and early medical intervention where necessary, islands can disappear and main lines be restored to strength and vigour, thus either preventing the development of disease or auguring a return to better health.

- A series of islands, better known as a **chain**, shows continued stress upon the constitution, thus undermining our general state of health. A fine tracery of links that break up the line half-way around its course may be linked to a deficiency of zinc.

- **Breaks** in the Life line need to be investigated carefully. Sometimes what appears to be a break might simply be the development of a new section of line, leading further out towards the centre of the palm (see Figure 50a). In this case, the marking suggests the beginning of a whole new way of life, one that takes its owner to new and wider horizons. A change of address or moving abroad may well, for example, be depicted in this way. Possessing this marking, then, can be a sign of expansion, of a new chapter in your life.

A true break, one that could be warning of an injury or of a life-threatening disease, is where an actual gap occurs in the line, an example of which is illustrated in Figure 50b. Discovery early enough and the right steps taken, can lead to the line mending itself before there is any real danger to the health.

There is a great difference between finding a broken line in the dominant hand as opposed to one in the passive hand. In the passive hand, a break denotes that the *possibility* of a major

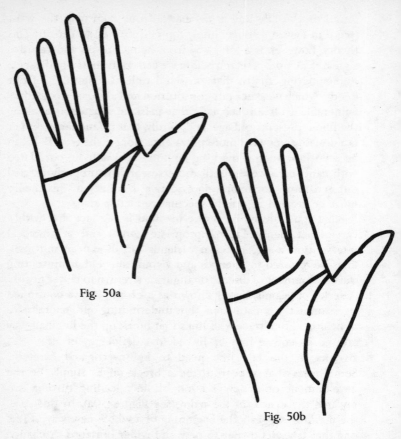

Fig. 50a

Fig. 50b

problem exists, whereas in the dominant hand, a break shows that the chances of either a serious accident or of the health severely breaking down are *that much more likely* to come about. More grave still is the situation where both hands possess the broken line at exactly the same location in each palm. Here, the message is clear and the odds stacked in favour of a breakdown in the health. If you find these markings in your hands you would be wise to take heed and take the necessary steps just as soon as you can to prevent the situation from happening.

Another factor to be taken into consideration here is whether the short Life line is overlapped by a new section with, very

Fig. 51a

Fig. 51b

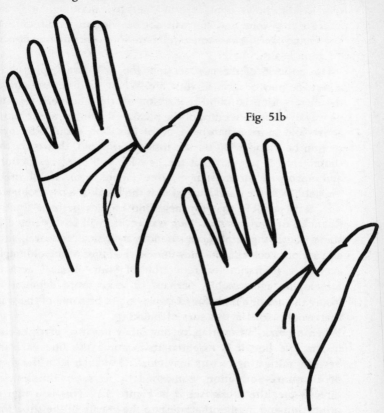

often, a fine hairline thread connecting the two (see Figure 51a). The overlapped lines are not as serious as the clean breaks but still, nevertheless, denote a break in the continuity and as such will represent a major change in the way of life. Other markings in the hand will throw light on the nature of the change, whether psychological (as with a move), or physiological (as in the case of accident or illness). What is important, if you possess this type of line, is to note the position and condition of the new section of line.

If the new section is strong and well-formed, you are likely to adapt well to your new circumstances and may even find that your new life is better than the old. But if the line is further islanded or shows signs of other negative markings, it could indicate that your new life will not be without its difficulties. The change, in this case, may well have some detrimental effects on your health.

The position of the new section, too, will give strong clues about the new chapter in your life. When, as discussed above, the new section is found to develop on the outside, sweeping its way towards the centre of the palm, it denotes a wider, more active and more expansive type of life. But, should the new section be found lying on the inside of the old, that is on the thumb side, it suggests that the new life will bring restrictions and narrowed circumstances, (see Figure 51b). If all other indications in the hand suggest that the break is a psychological one, it is possible that the new line implies perhaps limited finances, or perhaps that your way of life will be restricted in some way. If the implications denote a physical upheaval, such as a serious accident, the new line on the *inside* of the old might suggest a limitation or reduction of your physical activity. Developing agoraphobia, perhaps or, even more debilitating, losing the use of a limb, for example, might be some of the ways that would explain this sort of marking.

- When a break, an overlap, or any other negative mark occurs in the Life line it is essential to examine the line carefully because mitigating factors may exist. One such is in the form of a **square** formation, composed by four tiny lines, lying directly *over* the break (see *a* in Figure 52). This is a sign of protection and implies that, despite the gravity of the situation, the subject should make a full recovery.

- Another protective marking which is sometimes found is the **line of Mars** (see *b* in Figure 52). This is a line of varying length which is found on the inside (that is, on the thumb side) of the Life line and runs parallel to it, shadowing its course. Throughout its duration it represents a boost to the stamina and vitality of the individual so that if it occurs alongside a break in the Life line, or any other negative marking, it acts as an extra support, bolstering up the weakened constitution and shoring up the reserves. When looking at the health aspects in your hand, think of this marking as a secondary line of defence, or

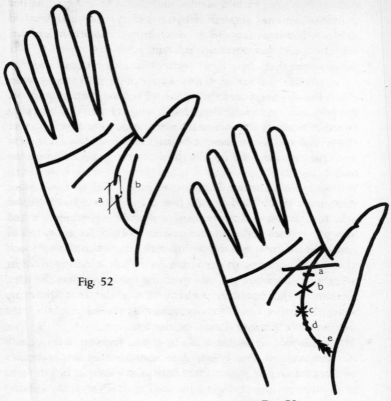

Fig. 52

Fig. 53

perhaps as the reserve parachute – just in case.

• Horizontal lines that cut across the main Life line are known
as **trauma lines** and denote a time of stress or emotional
upheaval, depending on the length and strength of the line. The
stronger and deeper the cross line, the more the effects will be
felt (see *a* in Figure 53). Similarly, the longer the line, sometimes
also cutting through the Fate, Head and Heart lines as well, the
greater the impact. Shorter, shallower crossing lines will suggest
that the interference is of a temporary nature and, given that
no adverse markings follow on the main line, the events should
not present any negative, long-term effects. A series of closely

packed fine lines should not be confused with the trauma line as these denote general hypersensitivity and highlight an anxious, highly-strung and nervous disposition rather than pinpointing an isolated traumatic event.

- Where two short bars form themselves into a **cross** over the main Life line, it is said to denote a time of physical danger when reserves of energy are being heavily drawn upon and are dangerously depleted. Some hand analysts see this marking, together with its sister-formation the **star**, as a warning of an illness that will require hospitalization and possibly even surgery. Both the cross and the star are illustrated at *b* and *c* respectively in Figure 53.

- A tiny indentation or **dot** in the line is said to represent a temporary shock to the body (see *d* in Figure 53). An illness which soon responds to treatment may be represented in this way but a series of these indentations, looking like a row of pinpricks in the line, may suggest that the nerves in the back and the spinal cord are under strain. A red or blue colouration, whether in the nails, the skin or in the lines, will alert the hand analyst to the circulatory system and a dot that shows up markedly red or blue is no exception as it could highlight the possibility of organic disease at the age indicated on the line.

- When the main Life line looks as if it is **fraying**, it suggests a draining away of energy which in turn lowers one's resistance to disease (see *e* in Figure 53). These lines must not be confused with the stronger single dropping branches that indicate movement and travel.

THE HEAD LINE

That our thoughts can generate tremendous power is succinctly put in the phrase 'mind over matter'. And when it comes to our health, we all know how easy it is to talk ourselves into feeling a good deal worse than we really are, or conversely, to cheer ourselves up when we're ill and consequently make ourselves feel better that much quicker. Our sensations and experiences of fear, anxiety or stress can all be intensified or reduced simply by our expectations, by how we think that a situation will affect us.

In the same way, we can control pain – indeed some are better at this than others. A fakir, for example, can lie on a bed of nails and get up again quite unscathed whilst you and I might howl and reach for the first-aid box if we merely prick our fingers with a sewing needle!

So our minds, then, have a powerful effect over our bodies and over our states of health. It is our minds, too – how we think and what we think about – that can trigger and release chemicals and hormones which are responsible for causing certain physical reactions in our bodies. And it is the action of these chemicals and hormones that can alter how well or how sick we are feeling.

Sexy thoughts, for instance, can stimulate the release of the hormone adrenaline which, amongst other effects, will dilate the pupils of the eye, quicken the heartbeat and send the blood pulsing through our veins. Endorphins, too, chemicals which are produced naturally in the brain can be released, when we hurt ourselves, and help to alleviate the pain in much the same way as a shot of morphine might.

With a positive attitude, then, we can help our bodies to heal themselves. Think negatively, and we open up our defences and make ourselves vulnerable to whatever disease is currently doing the round. So it is for this reason, because we have the mental ability to trigger and control our body chemistry, which in turn is responsible for altering our mood states, that our mental processes are so vital to our well-being. And these mental processes are registered in minute detail in our Head lines.

But this is not all, because the actual construction and composition of this critically important line will also give vital information on the mental health, the physical condition of the head and the brain together with any relevant details about genetic or congenital defects that might have been handed down. When piecing together clues about your health, then, a close examination of your Head line is essential because from it you can gather a veritable harvest of information which will throw direct light on how you cope with your health.

For a start, the actual direction and the path the line takes across your palm will reveal all sorts of things about how you think: whether you're the adventurous type, always prepared to experiment for yourself and try out new ideas, or whether you're the dyed-in-the-wool type, traditionalist, who takes a more practical and concrete point of view in all things. The way that you think about life and see the world around you will inevitably reflect your attitudes to your health and to your body in general, and will influence how you respond to disease.

The second part of the examination of the Head line must focus minutely and in detail on its texture and composition as well as on any markings or defects that may be found in the line itself. The condition of the line will give us specific information about susceptibilty to disease and psychological states of mind, highlight particular times of vulnerability and even give a fairly accurate idea of when the onset of any problem is likely to develop.

But, just as with all other main lines, the texture of the Head line should be compatible with the type of hand in which it occurs because a conflict would set up all sorts of tensions that would give rise to all manner of stress-related diseases. So a strong, fairly straight line would be expected on an Earth hand; a clear, distinct line with a springy curve in both the Air and Fire categories; but a much finer Head line and one that is more curved is suitable to the Water hand.

In general, the ideal Head line should be clear and well-etched, not too deep nor too shallow and it is best if it doesn't contain any defects or detrimental markings such as islands, breaks and crossbars. Such a line reflects an even temperament, an individual who is able to cope with the demands of modern life, with pressures at home and at work and who can take problems in her stride.

A wide and shallow line reflects a more diffuse way of coping with life's ups and downs. With one of these as your Head line, you would not be able to channel your energies so constructively. Indecision and a lack of concentration all too often are characteristic of this type of line.

A thin, wispy line, like a fine wire, is all too easily snapped. If you possess this type of Head line you should try to avoid taking on too much pressure because you can so easily buckle under the strain. Nervous exhaustion is always a threat with a fragile-looking Head line.

So the type, quality and condition of your Head line mirrors the way you think about yourself; reflects your temperament and your mental functioning; reveals both the psychological side, clearly depicting your different moods and mental states; and at the same time picks up on your physical condition, pointing out illnesses or injuries that could directly affect your head and your brain.

This is why the Head line is so valuable when it comes to building up a profile of your health. By understanding how you tick, by evaluating your attitudes and preconceptions, recognizing how you look at the world, by pin-pointing times of vulnerability, you may be able to change your outlook, to learn how to respond differently to situations which might otherwise have an adverse effect upon you, to change course and direction so as to avoid altogether those situations which physically present a potential threat to your health and safety.

Location: Working down from the fingers, the Head line is the second horizontal crease that cuts across the centre of the palm. In some hands it takes a straight course (see Figure 54a), almost as if it had been drawn in with a ruler, whilst in others it forms a gentle curve (see Figure 54b). In other hands still, the Head line slopes downwards sharply to end almost touching the wrist at the opposite edge of the palm (see Figure 54c). Sometimes the line may begin attached to the Life line (see Figure 55a) or perhaps begin its course from the mount of Mars (see Figure 55b) inside the Life line. At other times it may be found to take its root higher up in the palm, completely detached from the Life line and forming a wide gap between the two (see Figure 55c).

Psychological indications: The ideal beginning for a Head line is one that just touches the Life line or at least lies very slightly apart. This shows a well-balanced disposition, a healthy amount of self-confidence and a good ability to think for oneself. One that begins inside the Life line denotes an individual who tends to be clingy and dependent, who is cautious, timid, sensitive, anxious and withdrawn. Cautiousness, dependence and inhibition also applies to the Head line which is joined to the Life line for a long way, not breaking free until almost beneath the middle finger. People with this marking are said to be late developers. Beginning widely separated from the Life line, suggests a high degree of independence, adventurousness, dare-devil behaviour when young and a general recklessness, sometimes even foolhardy, tendency throughout life. The

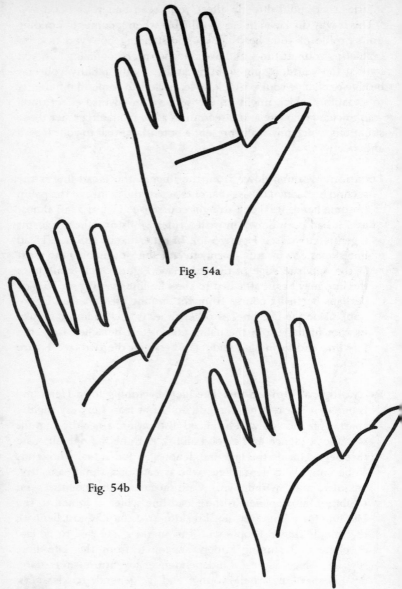

Fig. 54a

Fig. 54b

Fig. 54c

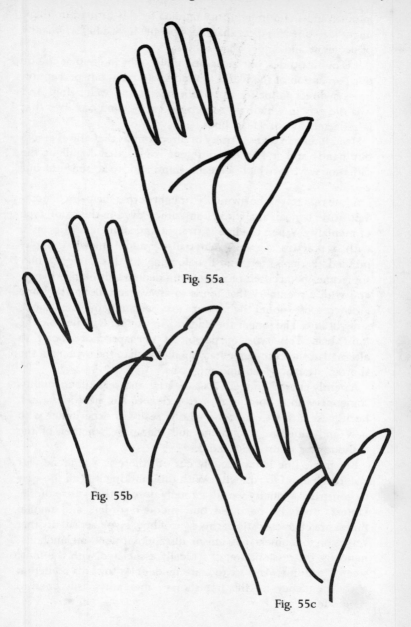

Fig. 55a

Fig. 55b

Fig. 55c

impulsiveness and impetuosity implied by this formation, then, might lead one to expect that these people have a higher chance of accident and injury than others.

It is our attitudes, our ideas, and philosophy in life that colour our perception of the world around us. In turn, our perception bears a direct influence upon our health and well-being. And it is the way in which we perceive ourselves and our lives that is reflected in our Head lines.

Head lines can take a variety of directions as they travel across our hands and it is these different routes that highlight the different ways in which we each think and make sense of our world.

A line that travels horizontally straight across the palm denotes a positive, logical, analytical, sometimes 'dyed-in-the-wool' type of mentality. When the line is straight and short it is associated with a practical person, materialistic and somewhat single-minded. Perhaps, too, those belonging to this category may sometimes be accused of narrow-mindedness, disliking change, and with a mentality that tends to always run along the same groove. Obsessional behaviour may accompany this short, straight line. The longer the line, the more mentally flexible the individual. This type of person is perhaps more open to alternative and complementary medicine than the owners of the shorter, straight Head line might be.

A gently curved line reflects a creative and versatile mentality, someone who is open to new experiences and new ideas and, healthwise at least, someone who is ready to experiment with new and different treatments and therapies, whether of the orthodox or unorthodox kind.

But if the line is too steeply curved, there is a tendency for the imagination to run wild. With this marking it is all too easy to construct a fantasy world, a totally unrealistic picture of life. Unless otherwise balanced out, mood disorders and mental illness are characteristic of this type of line. Hypersensitivity that verges on touchiness, pessimism, dissappointment, melancholia, neurosis, depression, are all typically associated with the long, steep Head line. And so, too, are tendencies towards addiction and dependency, for this line shows a mentality easily open to suggestion.

There are two exceptional forms of the Head line which bear distinct features and which have a specific bearing on mental health. The first is the Simian line (see Figure 56) and the second, the Sydney line (see Figure 57).

The **Simian line** is formed when the two lines of Heart and Head are joined together to form one solid crease that cuts horizontally across the centre of the hand, from one edge of the palm to the other. It is important to stress that the Simian line *is found in the hands of a small percentage of the normal population*, although it is a line that is more commonly associated with the hands of people with Down's Syndrome and other conditions caused by genetic defects and abnormal chromosomes. The distinction is that when the Simian line occurs in the abnormal hand, it is present amongst other unusual markings such as very short, pointed fingers, for example, small thumbs or displaced skin ridge patterns. All of these features make the hand instantly stand out as very different from the norm.

When the Simian line is found in a normal hand it denotes a strong-minded, determined and forceful personality, someone who possesses a restless, overactive mentality and who consequently finds it difficult to switch off and relax. Essentially, the Simian line is a sign of *mental and emotional intensity*. People with this marking often experience a conflict between their emotional feelings and their intellectual drives. In short, their hearts are at variance with their heads. And because of this, many show compulsive or obsessional behaviour in one form or another to a greater or lesser degree.

Their powers of concentration are so great that they can become totally single-minded, channelling their attention and focusing on only one activity at a time to the exclusion of all else. They have the power to absorb themselves so completely that they are able to screen out everything other than what they are doing, or feeling, at that particular moment in time.

Such intensity of purpose tends to rule their lives and their motivation in life. They are particularly highly achievement-motivated, with exremely high standards and even higher expectations, driving themselves hard to reach their objective and driving others just as relentlessly as they do themselves.

Simian folk function on extremes – everything is either black

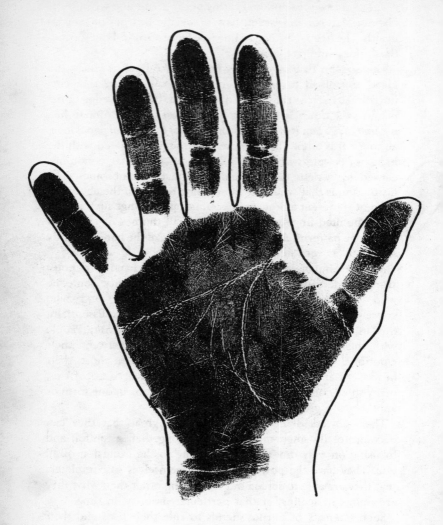

Fig. 56

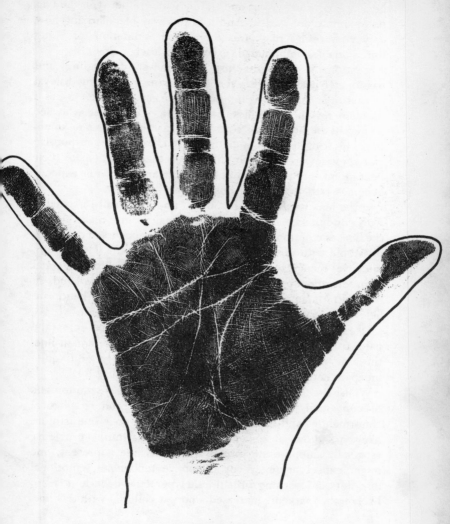

Fig. 57

or white, right or wrong, and sliding scales in between the two poles simply don't exist. And it is this way of polarizing how they view things that gives them their reputation for being unreasonable, opinionated, excessive in their demands.

Emotionally they are just as intense: demanding and passionately jealous if they feel their partners are being disloyal or that their affection is not being returned. And herein lies a problem for their families and working colleagues who see owners of the Simian line 'switching on and off', as it were, sometimes blowing hot and sometimes cold, sometimes responsive and sometimes completely distant, so that to anticipate their next mood and respond to it, as the Simian line owner expects, becomes rather a hit and miss affair.

In the abnormal hand, the Simian line is typically associated with conditions arising from an unusual genetic make-up and the line, as mentioned above, predominantly occurs in the hands of people with mongolism, or Down's Syndrome. Historically, midwives recognized that the marking was linked to congenital disorders and would immediately check for it in the hands of new-born infants. Figure 27, on page 67, is the handprint belonging to a 19-year-old Down's Syndrome sufferer.

Like the Simian line, the **Sydney line** also stretches across the palm from one edge to the other but, unlike the Simian line, this one is not fused with the Heart line but stands quite independently of it.

Whilst the Simian line in the abnormal hand is symptomatic of congenital problems that are likely to produce physical abnormalities and mental retardation, the Sydney line is more likely to show a tendency towards behavioural problems, especially amongst the young. When this line is present, one might expect aggressive or disruptive tendencies, emotional disorders and learning difficulties. Hyperactive behaviour is also likely to be markedly increased amongst children with this line.

Physiological indications: Apart from representing the psychological aspects, the Head line also registers the actual physical condition of the head, the skull, brains, neck and upper torso. Physical injuries, knocks and bangs, as well as diseases which affect these areas, fevers, headaches, dementia, paralysis or strokes, for example, will be marked on this line and discussed below in the section on specific markings.

Of the two special variants of the Head line, heart defects may be suspected when a Simian line is also accompanied by a complete set of arches on the fingertips and a displaced axial triradius pattern as discussed in Chapter 2. Indeed, the triradius on its own occurring higher up on the palm in the area governed by the Head line is enough to alert one's attention to cardiac problems, whether a Simian line is present or not.

In the case of the other unusual formation of the Head line, researchers have found that children with the Sydney line stand a greater chance of contracting childhood leukaemia than those with a normal line.

Length: Just as the length of your Life line is not an indicator of how long you are going to live, so the length of the Head line does not correlate to the level of your intelligence. It is the *texture* of the line – according to the type of hand in which it is found – and the *direction* which it takes across the palm that are both far more relevant to your IQ and, for that matter, that are important reflectors of your mental health.

SPECIFIC MARKINGS IN THE LINE

• **Islands** in the Head line can denote either a vulnerability to problems that affect the mental processes or a definite set period of worry and anxiety. Returning to the electric current analogy, remember that an island in the line splits the flow of energy and so reduces whatever power is at the individual's disposal. So, throughout the duration of an island in the Head line, the owner is not functioning mentally on all four pistons, as it were, decisions become noticeably difficult to make, and there is a good deal of woolly-mindedness and a marked lack of concentration.

In cases where the line begins attached to the Life line, islands may be present (see *a* in Figure 58) and these, as discussed in the section on the Life line, have two possible interpretations, one physical and one psychological. Either, they can denote susceptibility to bronchial and respiratory disorders, or they may represent problems and anxiety during the early years.

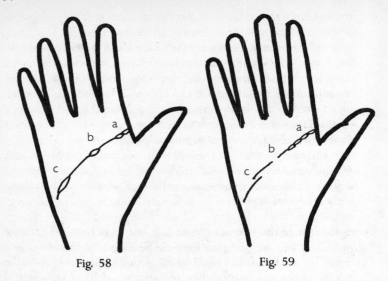

Fig. 58   Fig. 59

In some hands it is common to find an island half-way along
the Head line, directly beneath the middle finger (see *b* in Figure
58). Here the marking denotes that its owner finds it particularly
difficult to work under pressure. Some people fairly relish the
surge of adrenaline that a hectic, high-powered lifestyle
produces, but those with this type of island in their line don't.
They simply cannot function under stress and so need to learn
to pace themselves especially during such times as exams, say,
or when they need to meet a deadline; otherwise their health
will take its toll and they will end up mentally exhausted.

If an island is present towards the end of the Head line (see
c in Figure 58) it may represent the sort of mental conditions
that sometimes accompany old age. Forgetfulness, for example,
at one end of the scale, senile dementia at the other. Fears and
worries that beset the aged may also be denoted by the marking
in this position.

When an island is present in the Head line of the passive hand
but not in that of the dominant one, the source of the anxiety
is likely to be due to an emotional problem. Dissatisfaction with
personal relationships, unhappiness at home, marital problems,
for example. With this feature, a certain malaise is characteristic

but so subtle that often it is difficult to put one's finger on the problem. Though the problems don't actually manifest themselves overtly and the individual's thinking processes are not actually impaired, yet the dissatisfaction grumbles away in the background, niggling and gnawing at the back of that person's mind, permeating through and tingeing all other aspects of her life. Perhaps here the biggest problem is that of bottling up one's feelings, with all the attendant psychological disorders that this type of repression can bring in its train.

If an island is present in your Head line, it can be timed and will pin-point fairly accurately when your mental energy is likely to run at a low ebb, when you will be particularly undergoing a period of tension. A comparison with the other major lines will highlight the nature of the problem – perhaps it is related to dissatisfaction at work, if adverse markings are corroborated on your Fate line, or concerning an emotional upset if trauma lines are found across your Life line. And by working this out in advance, it is possible for you to plan a strategy to lessen the predicted effects of the stress, or even to find a way of avoiding the situation altogether.

- A **chained** Head line warns against overtaxing one's mental reserves because throughout the duration of the chained section, mental resources are at a low ebb (see *a* in Figure 59). During this time, too, because the thinking processes are weakened the owner tends to be more vulnerable to health troubles. It is possible that underlying this formation is a mineral imbalance in which case the diet might be investigated, as the sodium/potassium balance in the body could well be out of kilter.

- A clean **break** in the line, where there are no overlapping ends, may represent a physical injury to the head itself – a fall, an accident, or a blow for example (see *b* in Figure 59). Confirmation of such an event would be marked in the Life line at the corresponding time and, as with all such adverse markings, it is the construction of the line directly following the mark which reveals how the individual will respond to the situation. When the ends overlap (see *c* in Figure 59), is it unlikely that the marking refers to a physical event. More usually this would suggest a major psychological change of attitude and reorientation.

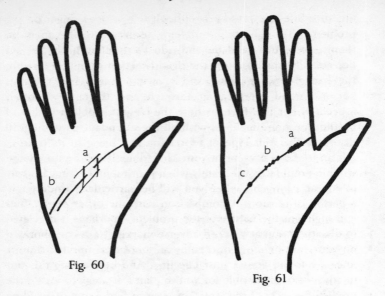

Fig. 60

Fig. 61

- Protection, or a form of secondary reinforcement, is represented by a variety of markings which appear over the defect on the line. A **square** formation, made up of four tiny lines over the break (see *a* in Figure 60) is one such protective feature and augurs well for a good recovery. Another sign with a similar meaning consists of a **sister line**, a small section of line that lies beside the fault and represents a shoring up of the energies (see *b* in Figure 60).

- A broad line with a **fluffy** or **fuzzy** appearance denotes a certain woolly-mindedness, an inability to make clear-cut decisions (see *a* in Figure 61). Here, the individual is not intellectually 'firing on all four pistons', is unable to think clearly perhaps because there is simply too much going on in his life at the time and he may be finding it difficult to cope with the demands placed upon him throughout the period marked on the line in this way.

  Quite often, rather than the whole line being broad and fluffy in this way, the fuzziness may appear in just one short section. It's common to see this, for example, in the part of the line that represents a woman's child-bearing years. Here, the fuzziness would equate to the draining effect that young, active children and a hectic family life has upon the mother. Alternatively, it might be seen later on in her hand during the menopause, say, when physical changes are taking place and hormonal activity is in a state of flux. During the time when the Head line is formed into this fluffiness, forgetfulness and tiredness are hazards to health, energies are being depleted and the constitution bearing the brunt. So, physical resources may slowly weaken and the individual becomes vulnerable to ill-health and disease.

- Tiny **indentations** like pin-pricks are a sign of a susceptibility to headaches and more particularly so to those of a migraine kind. Very often these appear in clusters, so denoting a time when a concentration of the problem occurs. If you can see a series of these little dots in your own line, but you don't as a rule suffer with migraine, the indentations may suggest sinus problems or catarrhal congestion that affects your head (see *b* in Figure 61). Or they may simply show that the condition runs in your family.

- A **dot** (see *c* in Figure 61) is like an isolated indentation and tells of an acute attack such as a dangerously high fever, perhaps, that temporarily affects the brain.

- A **dip** in the Head line, where along its course the line drops to form a tiny basin before regaining its normal direction, suggests a time of depression (see *a* in Figure 62). This is all the more emphasized if a small line sweeps out from the lowest point of the dip and shoots downwards. Using the timing gauge, the period when the depression is likely to set in, together with how long it is expected to last, can be measured and timed. Knowing of this possibility in advance may give its owner enough warning to be on the look-out for early symptoms and to deal with the situation before any ill-effects are felt.

- You will find some hands in which the Head lines form into a noticeable **zig-zag** as they travel across the palm (see *b* in Figure 62). This line as a whole represents a changeable, wavering, vacillating sort of mentality. Breaking it down into sections, it denotes periods of ups and downs, discreet phases of activity – constructive periods when the line rises and a lull when it falls. These switch-back periods can be accurately measured and timed by applying the timing gauge to the line. If, on the descent, the wavy line also forms itself into little dips it suggests that its owner has a tendency to slide into periodic spells of depression.

- **Crossbars** that cut the Head line suggest obstacles and set-backs

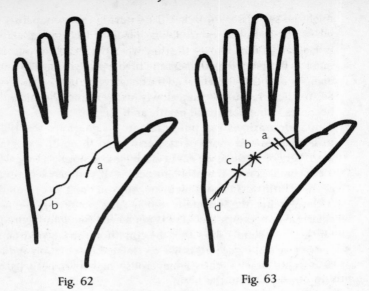

Fig. 62   Fig. 63

(see *a* in Figure 63). The implications denoted by these markings are likely to affect more the psychological well-being rather than representing a physical threat to the individual.

- A **star** formation, made up of several short bars that cross the line on the same spot is not a good sign as it tends to imply a shock to the system (see *b* in Figure 63). This may denote a psychological shock, receiving sudden and unexpected bad news, for example, or it might allude to a physical jolt, a serious bang on the head, perhaps, or graver still on the Head line, this might suggest a susceptibility to strokes. Whichever applies will be confirmed by other markings elsewhere in the hand, an island in the Fate line or crossbar cutting the Life line in the first case, or possibly a line connecting the star to a similar marking on the Heart line if the problem is an organic one. As with all such markings the section of line immediately following the star formation will highlight how the owner is likely to be mentally and physically affected by the event.

- A **cross** on the line will have the same meaning as the star, but only when it is clearly marked and deeply engraved (see *c* in Figure 63). The cross, however, must be made up of independent, free-standing lines and not by main lines, such as the Fate for instance, whose course will naturally take it over the Head line.

- **Fraying** towards the end of the Head line, giving the effect of a tassel, suggests mental impairment caused by a draining away of cerebral function (see *d* in Figure 63). Forgetfulness, senile dementia and Alzheimer's disease might all be represented in this way.

THE HEART LINE

The Heart line represents our emotions – how we feel about ourselves and about other people. On the psychological side, it reflects how we respond and relate to those around us, whilst physiologically, it reveals specific information about the circulatory and cardio-vascular system, about the heart itself as a physical organ and about the biochemistry of the body. As with all the lines, the dual aspects of the direction and of the formation of the line are as important as each other when it comes to building up a clinical profile of your health.

But when establishing the direction and location of the line, there is a division of thought amongst hand analysts about where the line actually begins, and this can be most confusing for readers, especially so for those who pick up the older books on the subject. The more traditional palmists and hand analysts believe that the Heart line begins beneath the index finger and swings out in the direction of the percussion edge of the hand. Others think the opposite, and believe that the line begins at the percussion and ends somewhere beneath the first two fingers.

In reasoning out the problem, perhaps matching up the characteristics of the other main lines to those of the Heart might help to solve the issue. For a start, then, given that in all hands both the Head and Life lines take their roots from more or less the same point, but may end in a variety of different places in the palm, seems to set the precedent and confirms the validity of saying that the Heart line begins under the little finger and not under the index. Moreover, the appearance of the Heart line at the percussion edge, with its width, its feathering and its often chained introduction, sweeping across to thin out towards the thumb side of the hand, would match the characteristics of both the beginnings and endings of the other two main lines. The argument, then, would logically support the belief that the Heart line does indeed take its root from the percussion.

From here the line travels across the palm and wherever it ends, whether beneath the middle finger, the index, straight across or up to touch the base of the digits, will give important insights into the way each one of us interacts with other people. But it is the construction and composition of this line, together with any defects or specific markings that might be found upon it, that registers the sort of health problems that directly concern the condition and functioning of the heart, the circulation and the blood vessels. And this information is mainly contained within the first four centimetres or so of the line where it passes beneath the little and ring fingers because this is the area that governs all to do with the heart and the lungs.

However, it must be emphasized here that **any negative indications in the Heart line must be backed up by other markings in the major lines or by other recognized features in the hand and fingers before drawing any conclusions or making any pronouncements about the owner's health**.

So, if you are looking at a person's hand and you think you may have spotted a defect in the Heart line, for heaven's sake don't jump to conclusions and frighten the living daylights out of your victim – even the most hardened sceptic has vulnerable moments. If you are truly concerned, advise the person to consult a doctor. Always remember: a) you might be quite wrong; b) the marking may be alluding to some emotional upset or psychological disappointment rather than to a clinical problem; or c) it may simply be denoting a predisposition to an illness and not to a fully fledged clinical or pathological development of disease.

The sort of markings that would accompany a susceptibility to cardio-vascular problems or to heart disease are well documented but vary from hand to hand and from person to person. In general, however, one might expect to find a bluish discolouration to the skin and particularly so at the base of the nails. Bulbous, or clubbed, fingertips, possibly with severely humped nails might also be present. Fan-shaped nails, too, are common signs of a tendency to circulatory problems. And so too are unusual fingerprints or displaced skin ridge-patterns such as a highly placed axial triradius for example, as discussed in Chapter 2. Severely malformed Heart lines, of course, would lead one to suspect damage due to genetic or congenital defects.

Location: The Heart line lies horizontally across the top of the palm and is the first line one encounters when working down from the fingers. It begins at the pecussion edge and sweeps out towards the thumb and terminates in a variety of ending points. Some lines are placed lower down than others, some are curved whilst others are straight. These differences in the location and course of the line distinguish the different ways that people feel and relate to others.

Psychological indications: The basic distinction between Heart lines is whether they are curved or straight. Their length and where they actually end will also give important psychological insights about the emotions.

- A **straight** Heart line denotes someone who is emotionally cool and undemonstrative, somewhat distant but very much in control of her emotions (see Figure 64a). A **curved** Heart line is quite

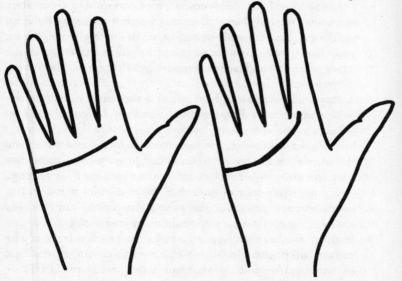

Fig. 64a   Fig. 64b

a different kettle of fish for this shows a warm and demonstrative lover, someone who is not afraid to wear her heart on her sleeve (see Figure 64b). When it comes to affairs of the Heart, the owner of the straight line may be characterized as emotionally passive whilst the one with the curved line is considered sexy and active in matters of love.

If you have a straight Heart line you will probably be very rational in your choice of partner, carefully weighing up the pros and cons of the relationship before committing yourself. Within the relationship, you will most likely want a strong mental understanding and indeed this aspect will be more important to you than the sexual, physical contact. If, however, you possess the curved line, emotional and sexual love will be essential as the basis to any relationship. You have to be physically turned on by your partner in order for you to commit yourself.

- A line **ending beneath the middle finger** is considered short and is found on those who crave sexual stimulation (see Figure 65a). In this hand the indications are clear – sex is more important than love, one-night-stands preferred to deeper, longer-lasting relationships. These people almost have an abhorrence of being 'tied down' or of committing themselves to another person. There is no true warmth of feeling here, no real love (except for oneself, that is), no desire to give or to share with anyone else. Unless modified by other markings in the hand, sensuality and personal sexual gratification are the driving instincts with this line.

- A Heart line that **ends high on the webbing between the first and second fingers** must naturally be curved and so belongs to the active lover category (see Figure 65b). With this line, however, although the disposition is loving and giving and the owner demonstrative towards her lover, yet she shows her affection through her actions rather than by voicing her feelings. If you have this type of line, then, you will find it difficult to verbalize your innermost feelings to the people you love. For you, the doing is more important than the saying.

- **Ending beneath the index, right in the middle of the mount of Jupiter** highlights the eternal romantic who sees everything through rose-tinted spectacles (see Figure 65c). There is an idealistic approach to love and relationships when this line

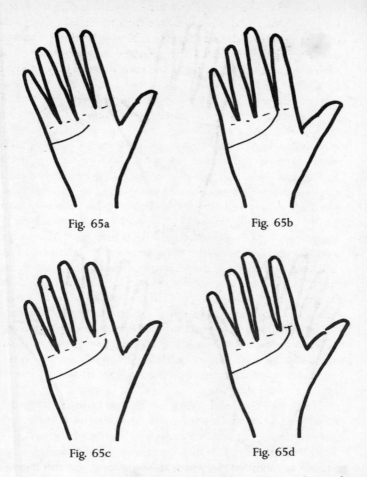

Fig. 65a   Fig. 65b

Fig. 65c   Fig. 65d

is present and unrealistic expectations about relationships. Owners of this type of line are often let down in relationships and matters of love simply because their ideals are unattainable.

- If the line reaches up and **touches the base of the index finger**, expect extremely high standards of excellence and even higher expectations in all relationships (see Figure 65d). If you are one of these you are a perfectionist, you drive yourself hard and expect others to do so as well. Possessiveness is one of your downfalls

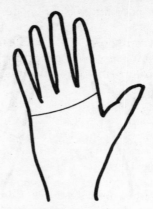

Fig. 65e

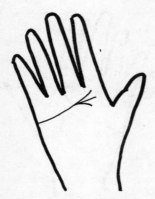

Fig. 65f

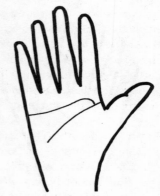

Fig. 65g

and, unless modified elsewhere in your hand, you can become
very jealous of those you love.
* People whose Heart lines travel **across the palm**, passing
  beneath the index mount to end almost touching the other edge,
  tend to have a vocational urge to care for others (see Figure 64e).
  Many of these people will be found on various committees,
  shouldering responsibilities, helping in the community. Others
  could simply be workaholics, putting their work and their jobs
  before their own emotional needs and those of their family.

- **Branched endings**, where the line splits into two or even three, shows a well-balanced attitude to emotions and relationships (see Figure 65f).
- A Heart line that turns down at its end and **falls onto the Head line** is the sign of a very sensitive nature, someone who gets easily hurt when love affairs and relationships go wrong (see Figure 65g).
- The **Simian line**, which is a thick crease that runs from edge to edge and which occurs when the Heart and Head lines have been fused together, is a special form of this line and has been fully described above in the section on the psychological indications of the Head line.

Physiological indications: Unusual formations and major deformities in the Heart line are associated with genetic and congenital problems and will often be found in the hands of people who are born with severe physical handicaps. Actual defects within the cardiac system or a susceptibility to heart disease may also be represented in this way or may be registered by negative markings occurring in the line beneath the ring and little fingers. However, as mentioned earlier, such formations would also be accompanied by other markings which would corroborate the situation.

Length: The length of the line in no way relates to longevity, and timing age and events on this line has been found to be unreliable. Markings such as islands and crossbars that occur in the line cannot be correlated in time but may be translated against the other major lines. In fact, quite often a bar or a fine line will connect a marking on the Heart line to one of the other main lines making it possible to assess the likely onset of the problem by timing the second line.

SPECIFIC MARKINGS IN THE LINE

- **Islands** occur naturally in most Heart lines as they enter the palm at the percussion edge. But if a single large island is found on the line either beneath the little or the ring fingers, and especially so if noticeably blue or reddish in colour, it may

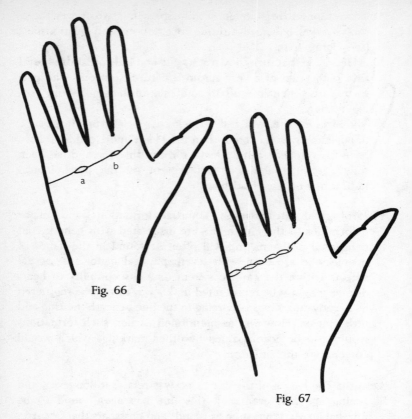

Fig. 66

Fig. 67

denote a susceptibility to heart disease (see *a* in Figure 66). Further along, a single island lying in the section of line that runs beneath the middle finger has been associated with hearing problems (see *b* in Figure 66).

• Psychologically, **chaining** or islanding in the Heart line suggests nervous or emotional tension and upsets. Physiologically, chaining that runs along for most of the length is associated with cardiac weaknesses and circulatory conditions such as irregularities in the rhythm of the heartbeat, palpitations and general erratic heart action (see Figure 67). Similar to the Head line, the chaining formation here may also suggest an imbalance of sodium and potassium.

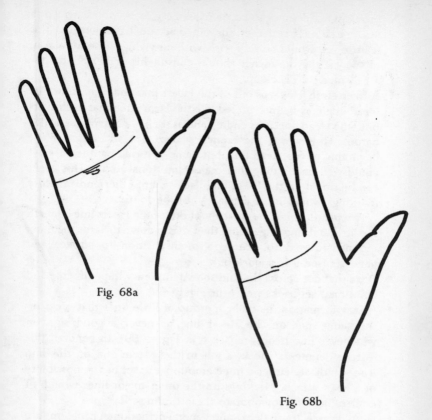

Fig. 68a

Fig. 68b

- Sometimes, a **ladder-like series of tiny lines** dropping from the Heart line directly beneath the ring finger is associated with a deficiency of calcium fluoride or with an imbalance of the calcium/magnesium levels (see Figure 68a). Insomnia, a change in the sleep pattern, anxiety and heightened nervousness may all be symptomatic of this deficiency.
- Just as with the other main lines, a **break** in the Heart line needs careful analysis, for here the marking can be very serious. If the line looks as if it has been snapped in two beneath the ring finger (see Figure 68b) and if there are corroborating features such as irregular skin ridge markings, cyanosis or blueness of the nails and/or fingertips, there could be some implicit cardio-vascular

problem, tendencies to coronary disease or even a danger of a heart attack. If you ever suspect that you have detected this feature you would be very wise, without giving cause for alarm, to suggest that its owner should consult his or her doctor for a full medical check-up.

- A **branch** that sweeps out of the Heart line and drops onto the Head line may be interpreted like the Heart line that itself wilts onto the Head line at its ending and as such is a sign of a sensitive nature. However, if the branch sweeps out and hits not the beginning of the Head line, but some point along its course, it could well be alluding to a major emotional upset. This event can be timed on the Head line itself where other confirmatory markings would most probably also be found.

  Two parallel branches that shoot out of the Heart line beneath the little and ring fingers and then sweep down towards the Luna mount are said to denote a predisposition to strokes and paralysis (see *a* in Figure 69).

- **Bars** that cut across the line show temporary impediments and emotional set-backs (see *b* in Figure 69).

- A **star** formation, made by a group of little lines that cross on the same spot on the Heart line, is never a good sign on whichever line it occurs (see *c* in Figure 69). In general, this feature denotes a shock, a jolt to the system and on this line it may indicate either a huge emotional upset or the possibility of a heart attack. Markings on the other major lines would, of course, have to corroborate these findings.

- Gum disease, tooth decay and general orthodontal problems are sometimes represented by a group of **tiny slanting lines** that lie just above the Heart line on the section that runs beneath the little finger (see *d* in Figure 69). Whether it is that in some cases gum disease is caused by stomach or liver dysfunction or conversely that such organic disorders can result in poor dentition is very much a chicken-and-egg situation. What has been found, however, is that the same group of lines that represent problems connected with the teeth and gums can equally reflect problems connected with the stomach, intestines and liver. But care must be taken when looking for these marks as they must not be confused with the Medical Stigmata, a larger formation of three oblique lines, often crossed horizontally by

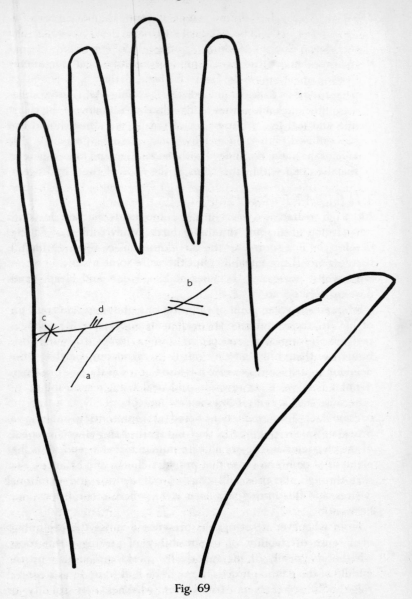

Fig. 69

a fourth, which in some hands is found higher up on the Mercury mount. The Medical Stigmata is discussed in the section on Special Markings on page 185.

- In some hands little hard lumps, or **nodules**, can sometimes develop on or around the Heart line beneath the ring finger either prior to a heart attack or immediately following one. These nodules are quite noticeable as they tend to distort the course of the Heart line and feel like a bumpy bit of scar tissue. They should not be confused with calluses which may often be present in this area of the palm, nor indeed with the tendons and knuckle bones that lie deep within the palm at the root of the ring finger.

THE FATE LINE

Although treated as a main line, in some hands the Fate line does not develop until some time after birth. Many babies, of course, develop the line soon after the three other major ones, during the first few months of foetal life. But there are some people, however, who, whilst possessing the lines of Life, Heart and Head, never develop a Fate line at all.

From an analytical point of view, the Fate line represents our way of life. It tracks and records movement and major life changes, registers information concerning our attitudes to our work, influences that enter and alter our lives, marks our sociability, our need for security and, because it is also known as the line of Saturn, denotes how we react towards, and deal with, responsibility.

Because it is a central line, it acts metaphorically as a fulcrum or stabilizer. It may be considered as representing an internal processing plant, pulling together and synthesizing all other aspects of the character and personality. In human terms it represents that element of common sense that provides checks and balances, that sifts through the pros and cons of our actions and emotional desires, and fills in the gaps, as it were, where other aspects may be wanting.

From whenever it springs, its presence denotes the beginnings of a sense of stability, of responsibility, of putting down roots, whether physically or metaphorically speaking. Running up the middle of the palm as it does, it might be looked upon as a central ridge pole so that its strength or weakness, its solidity or fragmentation, its degree of straightness or crookedness, corresponds to the amount of stability and good sense we feel we possess in life, and to the amount of security we want or are able to envelop ourselves in.

And the notion of the ridge pole also helps to explain the Fate line's other function, which from the medical point of view is so important, and that is its role as a support or supplement, principally to the Life line, but also to the other two lines of Head and Heart.

If, for instance, the Life line is patchy, or thin or adversely marked at any point, a strong Fate line at the corresponding time can bolster up any weaknesses implied and shore up a breach in our physical defences. Equally with the Head line, where a reciprocal relationship between the two exists. A patch of multiple Fate lines, for example, representing a frenetic burst of activity might find its correspondence in a fluffy stretch of Head line, denoting stress from over-work. Alternatively, a depression mark in the latter might highlight the results of an island in the former, suggesting that its owner's dissatisfaction at work during that time is a serious problem.

This is why it is essential that the lines in general need to be constantly cross-referenced, balanced off one with the other, compared and contrasted at every stage of analysis. And with none more so than the Fate line: this reflector and enlightener of events, this register of mental, physical and emotional detail, this supporter and sustainer, this central ridge pole upon which hangs a representation of our hopes and aspirations, our driving force, our ability to take charge and control of our lives and our destinies.

Location: Of all the lines, the Fate is somewhat of a maverick. It is read from the wrist up towards the fingers but it can have a variety of starting points in the palm and an equal variety of endings. Sometimes it may span the whole length of the palm, sometimes appearing only for a short while and then disappearing again altogether.

The line may take root from the very centre of the palm at the wrist, may begin attached to the Life line, originate from the mount of Luna or form itself from a number of locations further up the palm. Its designated ending is on the mount of Saturn, beneath the middle finger, although it may swing over to the

Jupiter mount, beneath the index, or the other way to end on the Apollo mount, beneath the ring finger. It may also peter out well before reaching the top of the palm or else come to rest at the Head line or terminate at the line of Heart.

Fortunately, the Fate line can be timed fairly accurately so starting and ending points in the line, as well as onset and duration of markings can be assessed with confidence.

Psychological indications: From a psychological point of view, the Fate line represents how much control we feel we have over our lives, over our immediate environment, over events that happen to us and over our personal destinies in life.

Personal control is essential to our psychological functioning, well-being, and peace of mind. If we feel we have the power to steer our own lives, to make our own decisions, to choose which way we want to go, we can maintain a buoyant outlook and a healthy state of mind. Take away our ability to make our own choices, take away any opportunity to shape our own lives for ourselves and we are stripped of our dignity, we become anxious, uncertain, dependent, depressed. Even the smallest modicum of personal control is enough to maintain interest, to keep a grip on life. Without it we lose motivation, we retreat inside ourselves and basically give up.

It is the Fate line in our hands, then, that registers the degree of control we feel we can exert. And it is from the very point in our palms that the line first appears that we feel we start to pick up the reins firmly in our own two hands.

The stronger the line appears, the more control we feel we have, the more we feel we can influence events around us. But strength, of course, is relative and the actual quality of the line must match the type of hand in which it is found otherwise conflicts within the personality may arise.

For the few who don't possess a Fate line at all, this doesn't necessarily mean a dull, uninteresting life. They can become as rich, as successful and as influential as the next person – as long as the other main lines are strong and well-formed, of course. But lacking this line can mean that its owner takes a non-conventional approach to life, does not care too much for commitment, for security or for laying down firm roots.

- A **strong** Fate line is usually found in the hands of people who
  have a good self-concept, a healthy amount of self-esteem and
  who understand their worth and standing in life (see Figure 70).
  People of good calibre might well be a fitting description for
  them. These people have plenty of drive, feel they can exert
  influence and are generally in control of their own lives. They
  are ambitious, make their own opportunities, possess the

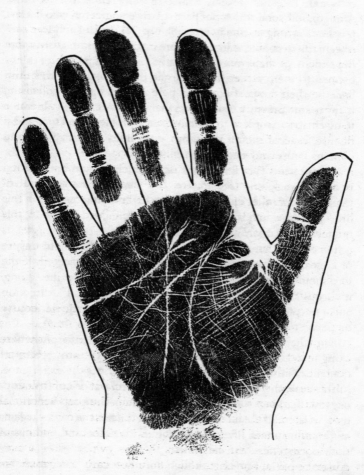

Fig. 70

capacity to succeed and achieve whatever goal they set their sights on. In all, they have strong and indomitable personalities with masses of will-power that can sustain any weaknesses that might appear in the other main lines. This type of line represents an excellent support system for any mental, emotional or physical problems that might arise.

- Just as a strong Fate line denotes a strong character, so a **faint or weak** Fate line reveals someone who tends to lack inner strength, someone who is not particularly resourceful, who doesn't possess a strong self-image (see Figure 71). With such low self-esteem, these people tend to be more emotionally immature, more dependent, perhaps more submissive, more inclined to let things happen to them rather than take the initiative themselves. And because their supporting 'ridge pole' is in danger of collapsing if any undue pressure is put upon them, they are more vulnerable to psychiatric disorders, to psychosomatic problems and to physical disease, especially so if the other main lines are also weak and contain faults and negative markings.

- A **fragmented** Fate line, one that is much broken and twisted is also a weak line (see Figure 72). There is a great deal of vacillation, of indecision, of stopping and starting implied in this line. In some hands the Fate line does indeed begin in this fragmented fashion and reveals a time when the youngster is trying to find her feet, perhaps going from job to job, unsure of a clear direction and as such possibly easily dejected. If the line should strengthen up and solidify at a point further along, it suggests that the individual does eventually find a direction and a purpose in life, and commits herself to a particular course or path.

  If an otherwise strong line breaks up into fragments somewhere along its course, it is likely that some event has 'thrown him off the rails'. 'Going to pieces' perhaps also describes the experience. In this case, the other lines should be checked for confirmatory negative markings such as depression, traumatic upsets, emotional upheavals, etc. If the line eventually mends itself, the owner regains her equilibrium in life. All beginnings, duration and endings of such occurrences can be timed.

- **Absence** of the Fate line, though not necessarily a negative sign in itself, may in some imply an unpredictable character and by

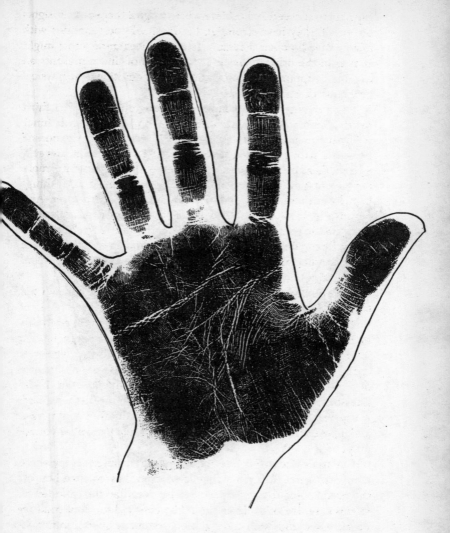

Fig. 71

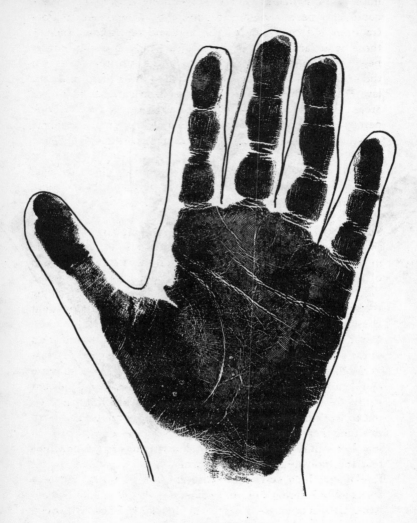

Fig. 72

implication someone who is not entirely trustworthy. There could also be a certain irresponsibility, a tendency to flout tradition and cock a snook at rules and regulations. Indeed, those who lack the line and whose hands also show other negative features may choose to make up the rules for themselves and some may even choose to live a life outside the law. From the little research that has been carried out in this area, there is some evidence for suggesting that a good percentage (although by no means all) of delinquents, and people showing psychopathic tendencies do not possess a Fate line.

It is the beginning and ending points of the Fate line that shed significant information about their owners' personalities and sense of well-being.

- **Starting from the centre of the palm at the wrist** and shooting straight up to Saturn denotes a solid, responsible individual with traditional values and a somewhat fatalistic turn of mind (see *a* in Figure 73). These people like to pre-plan everything they do in life, perhaps don't care much for taking risks and chances, and prefer the sort of life that others might consider unadventurous or stuck in a rut.
- **Beginning attached to the Life line** is a classical indication of early family responsibilities or duties (see *b* in Figure 73). Just as the line itself is tethered, as it were, to the Life line, so these people are tied to their families from a very early age, perhaps caring for a sick parent or having to leave school early and go out to work in order to support their families financially. With this line, there is a sense of restriction and dependency which may last well into adult life and colour any future relationships that the individual is likely to form.
- Fate lines which **start from the mount of Luna** denote a sociable and caring outlook, someone who is happiest when working with other people (see *c* in Figure 73). Those who need other people, who don't like being on their own, who enjoy life in the limelight, will invariably be found to possess this type of line.
- **Beginning further up in the palm** suggests that a true sense of purpose and stability are not achieved until a little later on

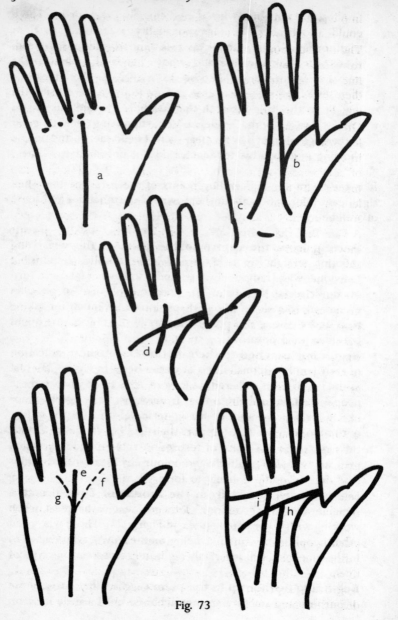

Fig. 73

in life (see *d* in Figure 73). This marking tells that success often comes to its owner in later years.

- The most common **ending for the Fate line is beneath the middle finger** (see *e* in Figure 73). Otherwise known as the line of Saturn, this is its most befitting destination, for the middle digit is called the finger of Saturn and the area beneath, upon which the line normally comes to rest, is the Saturn mount.

- One that **ends on the Jupiter mount** suggests a life and career led amongst people (see *f* in Figure 73). Those who care for others in the community and deal with the general public as a matter of course may possess this type of marking. For example, this line may be found in the hand of a doctor or local councillor, let's say, a popular figure, well-known amongst the people and someone who has achieved a certain standing in the community.

- A Fate line that swings over to **end on the Apollo mount** shows a turning towards a more creatively fulfilling way of life and thus one that promotes contentment and peace of mind (see *g* in Figure 73).

- **Ending on the Head line** has traditionally been described as implying that a major *faux pas* has been made that abruptly cuts its owner's career short (see *h* in Figure 73). In fact, this can simply suggest that one way of life, or one type of career gives way to another, especially so if the Sun or Apollo line is seen to continue on and take over. Healthwise, this could indeed be a most positive sign because as the Apollo line shows a sense of contentment and fulfilment, it would suggest that the new changes bring greater happiness and peace of mind.

- A similar meaning is ascribed to the Fate line if it should **end on the Heart line** (see *i* in Figure 73). Here, the traditional explanation given is that a major emotional blunder has terminated the career. But if similar markings to the above are present, what might at first appear as a negative outcome might, in fact, turn out to be a general improvement to its owner's well-being.

Physiological indications: Though not directly considered to reflect physical problems, the Fate line does act as a sister line to the Life line. It behaves as an insurance policy, so to speak. A strong line of Fate, then, will provide cover or shore up the defences where any breach or weakness in the Life line appears.

Length: Ideally, this line should stretch from the base of the palm right up to the base of the fingers, with no breaks or defects of any kind. But ideals aside, the Fate line may be found of any length, sometimes long, sometimes in short strands and sometimes missing altogether. Though this line can be measured and timed accurately, its length in no way equates with the longevity of its owner.

SPECIFIC MARKINGS IN THE LINE

Markings in the Fate line are significant for several reasons. Firstly, because this line represents our general way of life, any events, whether negative or positive, anything that is likely to affect the normal day-to-day running of our lives, such as a bout of ill-health, for example, will be registered here. Secondly, the Fate line acts as a support to the other main lines, and to the Life line in particular, so markings here will confirm and corroborate information gleaned elsewhere on the other major lines. And finally, this line can be timed with a very good degree of accuracy, which means that from it we can get a pretty good idea of both the onset and duration of events, states of mind, emotional reactions, or whatever, that may influence or disturb our daily lives.

The markings of greatest importance to the picture of our health consist of islands, chains, breaks, squares and stars.

- An **island** in the Fate line usually denotes a period of dissatisfaction and frustration whether with one's work or with life in general (see *a* in Figure 74). A period of financial difficulties and restrictions may also be represented by this formation. Whatever personal problem is being highlighted in this way should also be marked on the other main lines and in some cases is linked to them by a fine line as if directing attention to the very source.

- A **chained** formation weakens the line and thus loses its ability to prop up or support any of the other lines (see *b* in Figure 74). It is interpreted as a weak Fate line and as such has already been described above.

- A **break** in this line shows a change either in the workplace or in the domestic circumstances of the individual (see *a* in Figure 75). If it is a clean break, the change has been enforced.

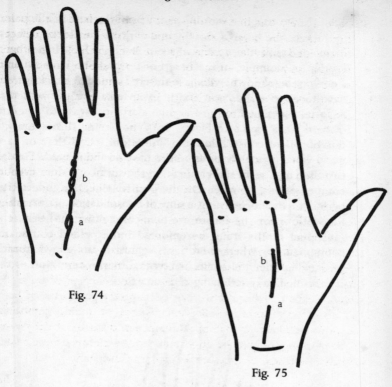

Fig. 74

Fig. 75

If the two ends overlap, the change is made at the owner's instigation (see *b* in Figure 75). For example, redundancy may be represented by the former, whilst applying for and getting a new job might well describe the latter feature. The condition of the line following the break as well as a comparison of the other lines for the same period is essential in establishing the effects that the changes may have upon the individual. Additionally, a break in the Fate line may not have the same impact on all types of people. People possessing the Earth and Fire hands, for example, might find the effects of a break more challenging, if not downright disruptive to their lives, than perhaps the Air or Water types who, because of their natures, seem more tolerant of change and variety.

- A **star** is invariably a warning sign when it occurs in a line and in the Fate line it can denote a time of crisis - a shock, perhaps, or major emotional upheaval (see *a* in Figure 76). It has been found, for example, in the hands of people who have suffered a nervous breakdown, who have suffered a sudden attack or who have received a dramatic and unexpected piece of bad news.

- A **square** attached to the Fate line alerts its owner to a period of hard work (see *b* in Figure 76). The feeling throughout its duration is of constriction and limitation. It is a time of hard grind when greater responsibilities have be shouldered. Though this time may seem rather bleak on the surface, it does have its compensations, however. On the positive side, this industrious period is a time of learning, a time of consolidation, a time when foundations for the future are being laid down. Whether the individual profits from the enforced industry and comes out triumphant, or whether he fights against it and allows himself to buckle under the strain, is revealed by the condition of the line immediately following the square.

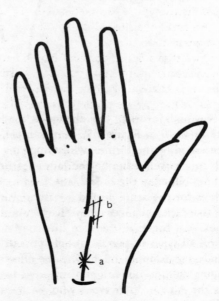

Fig. 76

THE HEALTH LINE

There is a good deal of confusion surrounding this line not in the least because historically it has been known by a variety of different names. The Liver line, the Via Hepatica, the Mercury line are just a few of its alternative titles, depending very much on which book on the subject you are likely to pick up.

Additionally, it may also be referred to as the Stomach or Spleen line and herein lies a clue as to its significance, because one of its major roles is to reflect the body's digestive functioning and eliminative processes. When these two functions are operating efficiently, the body is in a healthy state of being. But when digestion is sluggish, the whole system feels decidedly out of kilter.

Although the Health line is not always present in a hand, if you happen to possess one, it tells that you have a heightened awareness of your body mechanics. It shows that you are the sort of person who is conscious of every twinge, every ache, every heartbeat, every slightest change in temperature. Your Health line implies, in fact, that when it comes to the workings of your body, you are like a finely tuned instrument, a barometer perhaps, able to pick up and monitor, with fine precision, the state of your own health at any given moment in time.

Now, the fact that a house does not have a barometer in the hall doesn't mean for one minute that outside the atmospheric pressure is not subject to change. Weather systems will continue to form whether you or I are aware of them or not. The difference is that having a barometer hanging by the front door suggests that its owner *will* be alerted not only to current weather conditions, but will also be given some idea of what to expect next. Those who have a Health line have that health barometer built into their system. Those who don't have a Health line simply don't have that acuity, that sensitivity - they don't have that barometer to constantly remind them of what is going on inside their bodies. And, who can say, perhaps they are better off?

As any hand analyst worth his or her salt will tell you, lines can and do change and none more so than this line. In times of stress, for example, the line may be seen to grow and develop, sometimes longer, sometimes deeper. In times of ill-health, it might colour up a vivid red. Within a matter of days, the proper treatment, enough rest and even the smallest improvement to one's way of life can make an enormous difference to the whole condition of this line.

Location: The Health line, if it occurs at all in the hand, is normally found on the ulna side of the palm, that is, towards the percussion. It may take its root from a variety of places but in its more usual form it runs diagonally from the base of the palm up towards the little finger (see Figure 77). In some hands it may strike the Life line, in others it may cut through this line and run into the mount of Venus. In others again it may shoot up from the mount of Luna. Sometimes it is a whole line stretching the whole length of the palm from base to fingers. At other times it may exist only in short stretches located anywhere between those two points.

Psychological indications: The Health line is perhaps more valuable as an indicator of physical disorders rather than as a reflector of the psychological state. But, having said that, when we aren't feeling physically well we're unlikely to want to dance

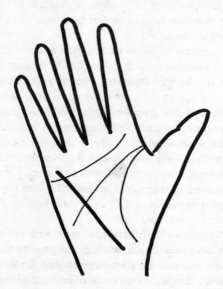

Fig. 77

and cheer. Pain and discomfort will usually make us feel crabby and miserable. Enthusiasm will be at a low ebb and our outlook somewhat bleak. So a poorly formed Health line, whilst representing physiological disorders, will also inevitably reflect the sort of state of mind that accompanies ill-health.

Additionally, because acidity, ulcers, indigestion and general gastric conditions may be caused by nervous tension, the Health line can be consulted for corroboration of nervous fatigue or stress-related problems, which are first picked up on the other main lines.

Physiological indications: Most hand analysts agree that the best Health line to possess is, in fact, no Health line at all. In so far as a line in the palm denotes an awareness of whatever that line is representing – that is, the Head line reflects our mental or intellectual awareness, the Heart line our emotional awareness, etc. – the Health line then, by definition, highlights our awareness of the state of our health. So for this reason, you could argue, *not* possessing this line is perhaps better for us than possessing it.

But if we must have one, then it is judged far better to have a strong, long and unblemished line. Such a line reflects a robust constitution, plenty of vitality and a good ability to keep illness and disease at bay. A good, clear line also suggests that the metabolism is in good order and the immune system is functioning efficiently. Any defects, markings, twisting or fragmentation of the line, however, all imply potential health problems with each marking denoting a susceptibility to a particular physical illnesses.

Health problems which may variously be represented by this line include intestinal and digestive disorders, kidney and liver dysfunction, respiratory ailments and problems of the gynaecological system.

Length: The line varies in length from hand to hand and does not equate with longevity. Illnesses which may be marked in the line will be found to have their corresponding signs on the other major lines, in the Life line in particular, and may be timed accordingly there.

SPECIFIC MARKINGS IN THE LINE

Although a defective Health line will give us a fair idea that our systems are under stress, actual defects and markings in this line are not necessarily specific to particular organs or their diseases. In broad general terms, the markings here suggest that something is going wrong, that some organ or other is not functioning as it should or that there is a strong vulnerability to certain disorders.

Most of the markings will be found in some way or other to suggest some dysfunction in the organs of digestion and elimination but for greater accuracy any markings that may occur can usually be found to have their counterpart somewhere else in the hand, and principally so in the other main lines.

Despite this, however, some of the markings do have traditional associations and these will be given below wherever they apply.

- **Islands** in the line, as with all islands, show a period when the constitution is running at a low ebb (see *a* in Figure 78). They

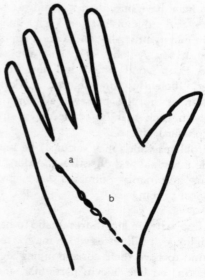

Fig. 78

can also represent the actual duration of an illness. In addition, islands in the Health line have a traditional association with a predisposition to chest infections and general problems of the respiratory system.

- A **chained line** will indicate general debility and a weakened constitution (see *b* in Figure 78). Perhaps this formation may also suggest that the immune system is under stress.
- A **twisted or wavy line** is normally associated with stomach, liver, gall bladder or intestinal problems (see Figure 79). Dyspepsia and other digestive complaints may be represented in this way and especially so if the line itself begins on the mount of Venus inside the Life line.
- A **broken Health line** or one that is much fragmented is often a sign of ill-health; the aspect which is particularly under stress will be marked elsewhere (see Figure 80). The broken Health line can also indicate problems connected with the stomach and liver.
- Again, the sound functioning of the stomach and liver comes into question when the line is much fragmented so that it forms

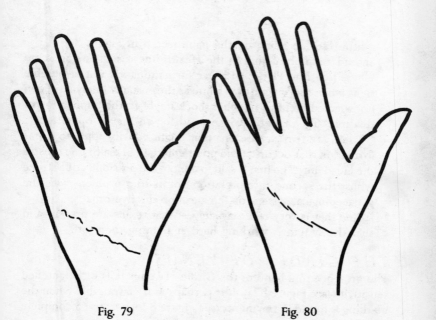

Fig. 79   Fig. 80

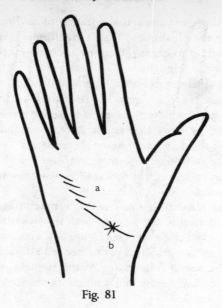

Fig. 81

a little **ladder** rising up the palm (see *a* in Figure 81).

- Should a **star** be found in the Health line it suggests an acute illness (see *b* in Figure 81). Star formations are not favourable signs when they occur over a line as they usually imply a sudden unexpected event. A possible shock might fit the implication of this marking, or perhaps the need for an urgent operation.

  There are two suggestions that might equally apply to a star formation that occurs at the point where the Health line crosses the Head line. The first is said to denote the possibility of a stroke whilst the second interpretation points to a problem with the gynaecological system or female reproductive organs.

- A line that is very **red** may suggest that toxins are present and that the system is working hard at fighting them off.

THE GIRDLE OF VENUS

The presence in a hand of the Girdle of Venus tells of heightened sensitivity (see Figure 82a). It is perhaps more favourable when the marking is found in fragments (see Figure 82b) because a complete

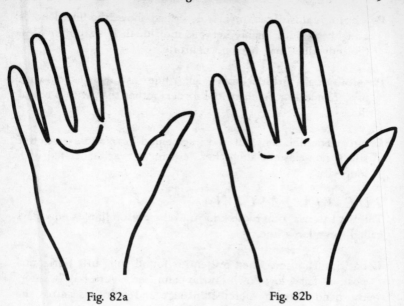

Fig. 82a   Fig. 82b

semi-circle denotes an individual who is especially nervous and, in extreme cases, someone who is susceptible to neurosis.

People possessing this marking are generally highly imaginative types and, whilst an excellent sign for a creative turn of mind, when it comes to health there is a tendency to turn that imagination inwards so that dark brooding, unhealthy obsessions and a tendency towards hypochondria results. Thus it is that people with the Girdle of Venus imagine that they have every disease in the book. And many go so far as to convince themselves that they are ill to the very point where they actually suffer with a wide range of psychosomatic ailments.

Location: In its most prominent form, the Girdle of Venus is a semi-circular line found at the top of the hand between the Heart line and the base of the fingers. It enters the palm from the webbing beween the first two fingers and sweeps its way across and up to end on the web between the ring and little fingers.

Psychological indications: As described above, the line denotes a highly anxious, highly nervous individual. In extreme cases, the individual may become neurotic.

Physiological indications: The line is associated with psychological or psychiatric disorders rather than with physical illnesses.

Length: The line is best if in a fragmented form and even better still if non-existent altogether. It is in no way associated with longevity.

THE VIA LASCIVIA

The Via Lascivia, otherwise known as the poison line, is nowadays called the allergy line.

Location: The line, when present, is found lying in a horizontal position fairly low down on the palm (see Figure 83). It enters the hand from the percussion edge and proceeds across the mount of Luna towards the Life line.

Psychological indications: Psychologically, the line is associated with hyperactivity for it is often found in the hands of children who display hyperactive behaviour. It is also often found in the hands of addicts.

Physiological indications: Known as the allergy line, when present it denotes a delicate physiological system, one that is especially sensitive to drugs, chemicals, airborne pollutants, alcohol, nicotine and various other types of allergens. The line, however, simply suggests that a sensitivity exists; it does not, unfortunately, highlight what the body is actually allergic to. In order to find that out, the owners could perhaps keep records of their diet and nutrition and carefully note any chemicals they come into contact with, together with their reactions. In serious cases, a desensitization programme or an elimination or detoxification diet might also prove useful as long as these are carefully monitored by medical practitioners or professional dietitians.

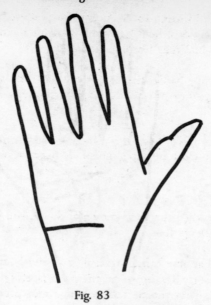

Fig. 83

In view of their sensitivities, homoeopathy is perhaps more suitable for these people than the harsher types of allopathic medicine.

SPECIAL MARKINGS

TRAUMA LINES

Heavy lines that cut right across the Life line are known as trauma lines and denote times of emotional upset. The gravity of the situation is very much reflected by the depth and length of the line. The more serious the upset, the thicker and longer the crossbar, sometimes cutting through the other main lines of Head and Heart as well. Any consequences of the disturbance may be echoed by corresponding markings in the other main lines, and also by the condition of the Life line immediately beneath the point where the trauma line crosses. An island in the line, for example, would suggest that the event has set up a reaction which would last for some time, having perhaps unsettled the individual's health.

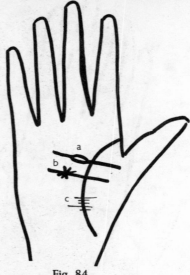

Fig. 84

- If an island should occur in the line itself, the worry may concern some aspect of the health (see *a* in Figure 84).
- A star on the crossline would denote a shock of some kind (see *b* in Figure 84).
- A series of very fine lines that cross the Life line are not considered to be trauma lines. Such lines merely denote a nervous, highly-strung disposition (see *c* in Figure 84).
- Trauma lines can be measured and timed against the Life line at the point where they cross. This could well give the individual enough warning to take preventive measures and avert the situation.
- Trauma lines that denote an intense period of tension and worry can be made to disappear often by taking a more relaxed view, by changing one's attitude, reviewing the diet, etc.

VEILING ON THE PERCUSSION
When the area around the edge of the palm beneath the Heart line appears heavily criss-crossed by fine lines, as in Figure 85, it is

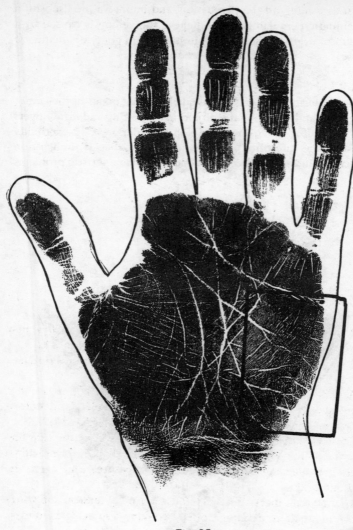

Fig. 85

known as 'veiling on the percussion' and implies a predisposition
to rheumatic complaints. Some believe the veiling is caused by a
build-up of uric acid, sometimes implicated in gouty or rheumatic
illnesses.

FLARING

Flaring is a term used for fine oblique lines that occur in the centre
of the palm and rise up in the direction of the ring and little fingers
(see Figure 86). When these develop they denote a susceptibility
to gastric and intestinal problems. Acidity, dyspepsia, indigestion
and general intestinal discomfort could be characteristic problems

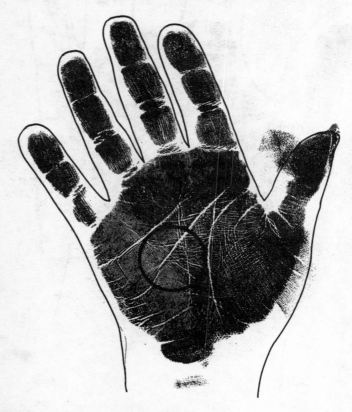

Fig. 86

for those possessing the marking. A poor diet could well be the underlying cause here but so too can anxiety.

HORIZONTAL LINES ON FINGERTIPS

Sometimes called white lines, horizontal dashes found across the fingertips are one of the first signs of stress and worry (see Figure 87). These are some of the fastest lines to appear and disappear again as tension is built up and then released again. Sometimes they

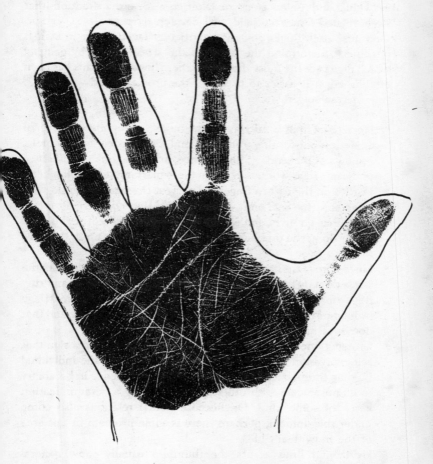

Fig. 87

can come and go within a matter of days and sometimes they remain - a witness to the fact that the problems are as yet unresolved - for several years. Pre-exam tensions may well cause some of these lines to develop as well as, say, unhappiness due to a marriage break-down. In some cases, a few random lines may appear on the odd fingertip but, in others, so many lines may develop as to almost obscure the ridge-pattern on the finger. When this occurs it is a warning that the problems are overwhelming the individual and, unless steps are taken to resolve the situation, that stress-related illnesses could well develop.

Because each finger governs a particular facet of our lives, it is possible to determine the cause of the stress simply by gauging which digits are the most affected by these lines. Once this has been established, it is easier to tease out the problems and work out a way of resolving them.

- Horizontal lines occurring on the index often point to personal anxieties concerning one's general confidence and morale. Feelings of inadequacy, for instance, or having one's confidence undermined at work, may cause these markings to develop here.
- Dashes on the Saturn fingertips suggest that matters to do with one's security and one's home are causing concern. Property deals that go awry, for example, may be reflected in this way. Other domestic problems and worries may show up in this way, too.
- Lines across the tip of the ring finger usually denote that the stress directly involves a relationship. If both the middle and ring fingertips are equally marked in this way, suspect that a marriage or long-term partnership is going through a stormy time and that domestic harmony and security are under threat.
- Crossing lines on the tip of the little finger are often a sign that self-expression is presenting a problem. Perhaps the individual is going through a period when he lacks confidence in his ability to communicate with others, or is suffering a communication block of some kind. Or, because sexual relations also come under this domain, perhaps there is some problem in this area of the individual's life.
- Horizontal lines across the thumbtip usually show general nervous strain. When these occur it is a sign that some kind

of stress-management strategies should be found and put into operation. Perhaps some form of meditation, yoga or deep-breathing relaxation techniques might prove helpful in these cases.

VERTICAL LINES ON FINGERTIPS

Although more research is required in this area, evidence suggests that there is a relationship between the fingertips and the endocrine system. Each finger, it is believed, is linked to a particular gland so that the condition of that gland is mirrored on its corresponding tip.

Glands of the endocrine system produce and release hormones which are absorbed into the bloodstream. These hormones either cause vital chemical changes themselves or act as a cue to other glands, triggering them into activity. Like a well-tuned engine, every part of a healthy, well-balanced glandular system will secrete the correct amount of hormone according to the body's needs, and in turn will send the correct messages to other glands to prompt them into action. But, should a gland malfunction, should it become diseased and produce either too much or too little secretion, the balance will be upset and the chain reaction will go awry.

It is this very malfunctioning or disturbance of a gland that is reflected by vertical lines that run up from the top joint of its corresponding finger (see Figure 88). These lines must not be confused with the stress and tension markings which run *horizontally* across the fingertips. It is specifically the *vertical* lines that are associated with an imbalance in the workings of the glands.

The increasing evidence that is now filtering through to us from the ancient practices of acupuncture, reflexology and shiatsu does indeed seem to confirm a relationship between our internal organs and their corresponding external links. These practices have been in operation for thousands of years and the external terminal points of organs and glands are well established. But in hand analysis, evidence of these connections has started to be gathered only comparatively recently and no one would dispute the fact that a good deal more research in this area needs to be done.

So far, our understanding of the connections suggests the following linkage:

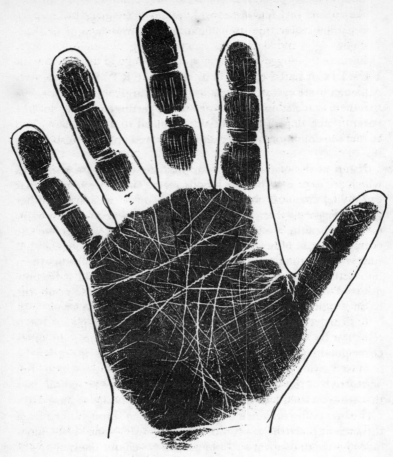

Fig. 88

- The fingertip of the index is believed to correspond to the pituitary gland. Of all the glands in the endocrine system, the pituitary is the most important for it produces and releases several essential hormones which control the activity of many other glands in the system. Interestingly, reflexology places the pituitary link in the thumb.

- The tip of the middle finger is said to be linked to the pineal. We don't as yet know the exact function of this gland but suspect it plays a major role in maintaining our awareness of day and night, light and dark, and in controlling our daily rhythms. Because this suggests that the pineal has a good deal to do with the maintenance of the body's balance, it would seem well placed here on the Saturn fingertip as this digit corresponds to our sense of stabilization. Reflexology, however, sites the gland's terminal point, like that of the pituitary, in the thumbtip.

- The tip of the ring finger is said to be associated with the thymus, a gland which plays a major role in the immunological system. However, because the ring finger and area on the palm directly below it are associated with the heart and the circulation, it would seem more logical that vertical lines on this tip should be reflecting some malfunction of the cardio-vascular system. Although this hypothesis is highly speculative at present, it is interesting to note that people with hypertension, or high blood pressure, have also been found to possess heavily lined tips to their third fingers. Interesting, too, is the fact that in reflexology the thymus link is found on the palm in a line directly beneath the ring finger. The function of the thymus has been obscure until recently and it is only since the 1960s that we have come to realize the vital policing role that it plays in the immune mechanism. Given the coincidence that hand analysts see between this gland and the area in the hand that represents the heart, who knows, perhaps in time medical researchers will establish a link between the thymus and the circulation system, too?

- The little fingertip is connected with the thyroid gland and much evidence would suggest that this is indeed so. Vertical lines here can indicate over- or under-activity of the gland, producing either too much or too little thyroxine, the hormone responsible for regulating metabolism. An imbalance of iodine, central to the production of the hormone, may be suspected in certain cases when the gland is defective. Action of the thyroid gland is triggered by the pituitary.

- The thumb has not as yet had a glandular connection ascribed to it. In hand analysis, this top phalanx of the digit reflects our will power, the power of our mental control over all other aspects in our lives. Isn't it interesting, then, that reflexology should recognize a connection between this area and the pituitary, the master gland that controls the activity of so many other glands in the endocrine system? Reflexology also sites the pineal here, and as both these glands are indeed located in the brain, perhaps it would be more logical in the thumbtip (that is, from the point of view of hand analysis, that both glands should find their correspondence at the seat of mental control), rather than on the tips of the middle and index fingers as is currently thought by many hand analysts today.

It is evident, then, that although a lot of valuable work has already been carried out, and has got the research going, a great deal more has to be done in order to identify correctly the glandular links. And yet, there is still a good deal of justification in accepting that the vertical markings on the fingertips do correspond to stressed or malfunctioning glands even if, in some cases, we haven't quite got the right finger on the right button yet.

TIREDNESS LINES
Tell-tale signs of tiredness may be seen as strong vertical lines that run up the two basal phalanges of the fingers (see Figure 89). When many of these lines are seen they are a warning that the body is nearing exhaustion and needs time to rest.

DIAMOND OR TRIANGULAR FORMATION
A group of lines that form themselves into either a diamond or a triangular shape attached to the Life line, as shown in Figure 90, often suggest a susceptibility to problems of the reproductive organs in women, and the uro-genital organs in men. Emphasis must be placed on *susceptibility*, as many women who have the marking don't necessarily develop any clinical complications. If problems were to develop, other markings, such as stars or islands in the appropriate place on the Life or Head lines, would also be present. The sort of health problems associated with these patterns might range from irregular menstrual cycles to the need for a hysterectomy in women. In men, similar markings might suggest a tendency to hernia, whether congenital or acquired, or perhaps diseases affecting the testes or the urological system in general.

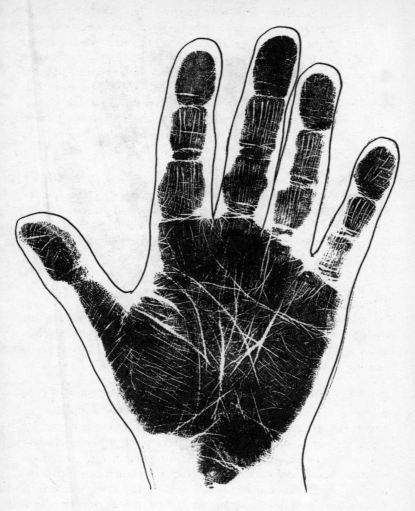

Fig. 89

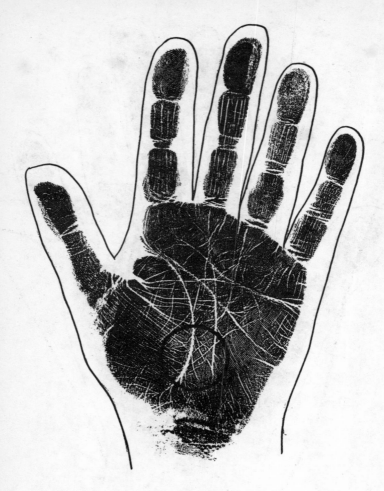

Fig. 90

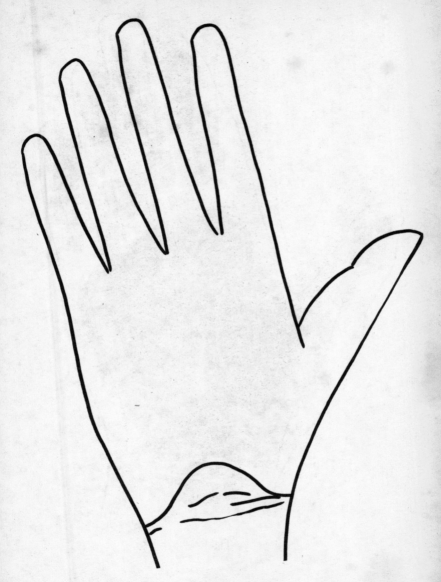

Fig. 91

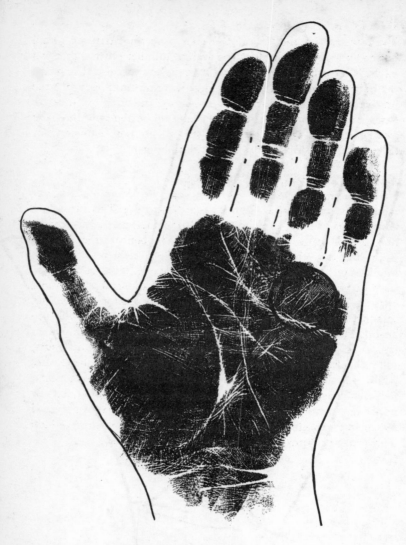

Fig. 92

DISTORTED RASCETTES

The rascettes are the 'bracelet' markings or rings that are found on the wrist, (see Figure 91). The average number of rings that you might possess is about three and it is the top rascette that forms the boundary between the hand and the arm. On most arms, the bracelets form a neat horizontal line across the wrist but in some cases, the top ring is distorted and visibly arches up onto the palm (see Figure 91a). When this occurs it is a sign that its owner may have a predisposition to problems in childbirth.

THE MEDICAL STIGMATA

No discussion on health markings can be complete without mention of the Medical Stigmata (see Figure 92). This formation is made up of three oblique lines with, sometimes, one crossing line, and is located high on the palm directly beneath the ring and little fingers. When present, the marking reflects a natural, inherent gift for healing. It tells of a wonderful 'bedside manner', a sympathetic way of dealing with others. Not all medical personnel possess the marking but those who do stand out for their ability to empathize with their patients. It may occur in people who use healing in the unorthodox fields too, amongst practitioners in fringe or complementary medicine – osteopaths, masseurs, reflexologists, for example. And it may also be found in those who, whilst not medically qualified, work in the caring or vocational fields, such as counsellors and psychologists. But, whether actively in healing or not, anyone with this marking will possess a natural reassuring, soothing and therapeutic quality about them which seems magically to rub off on those around them.

4

Reflexology

PRESSURE POINTS

The art of reflexology has been practised in the East for thousands of years and was introduced into the West in the early part of this century by an American doctor, William Fitzgerald. Although in existence for centuries, in one form or another, no logical scientific explanation has yet been found to explain satisfactorily how or why it works. That it does work, however, is to reflexologists indisputable, the majority of whom will readily provide personal anecdotal evidence in support of its claims as a system for diagnosis and as an aid to healing.

The underlying principle of reflexology is based on the theory that a link exists between, at one end, the muscles and organs inside our bodies and, at the other, terminal endings which are located in our feet, in our hands and in our ears. In reflexology, the body is divided off into ten areas with a midpoint line running vertically down the centre, five zones on either side of the line, each connected to specific points on the terminal extremities.

Particular muscles or organs correspond to these specific, or reflex, points on our feet, hands and ears so that any upset at one end of the link will produce a related effect at the other end. For example, a pain in your lungs would present some discomfort in its corresponding area on the sole of your foot, which in this case lies a little way below your fourth toe. Working the other way around, massaging this area has a direct stimulating and therapeutic effect on your lungs and bronchial regions.

Under this system, all the organs within a zone are interrelated one with another, so if an imbalance or a break-down should occur in any of these organs, the others in the same zone may be affected, too. By massaging or applying pressure to the corresponding point on the hand, foot or ear, then all the organs within that same zone will subsequently be affected. The five zones on the left side of your body find their reflex points in your left foot, hand and ear, whilst those on your right have their corresponding connections in the right extremities.

The massaging technique in reflexology is quite specific and the method used consists of applying direct, though not too firm, pressure with the thumbtip to particular points, pressing down on the spot with a circular motion. Any reaction that is felt – a referred tingling sensation or sharp stabbing pain – suggests a problem or imbalance in its corresponding vital organ. By massaging that point it is possible directly to stimulate the organ into eliminating toxins from the body, redressing that balance so that the normal chemical equilibrium of the system is restored and thereby aiding not only the organ to heal itself, but also encouraging the natural healing process *throughout* the body to take place.

Although no one would claim that reflexology is a substitute for conventional medicine, recognizing the location of the reflex points in our hands and feet and understanding how the pressure technique works means that we may be able to regulate stress, ease headaches, relieve backache, combat fatigue, control weight and generally tone up our nervous systems. Thus reflexology teaches us that pain, tension and disease can be prevented and literally rubbed away by daily massaging, and by doing this we will be promoting and enhancing both our physical and psychological well-being.

Whilst in reflexology it is the foot that a practitioner will concentrate upon, the hand is no less sensitive and receptive to this type of pressure massage and, from a chirological point of view of course, it is more appropriate. One of the benefits of working on our hands is that we can carry out a programme of massage quite unobtrusively wherever we happen to be, whether in public or in private. Another benefit is that, although it is perhaps more comfortable and more relaxing to be treated by someone else, at least working on our hands is fairly easy to do for ourselves, using the thumb of one hand to massage the other hand.

But whether using the technique on your hand or your foot, you must first take into account whether you have any specific medical conditions, because the massaging of some of the parts is not recommended in certain circumstances such as pregnancy, for example, or with particular types of cancer, and especially not after surgery.

REFLEX POINTS ON THE HAND

Figure 93 illustrates the position of the reflex points in your hands that connect with the muscles and vital organs in your body. Essential differences occur between your right and left, according to the zone in which an organ is situated. Your heart and liver are particular examples, the liver being situated on the right side of your body midline and the heart on the left. When the muscles or organs come in pairs, such as your legs, kidneys or ovaries, each will correspond to the terminal ending on its appropriate side. Equally, when the organs are found down your central midline, they, too, will be connected to both hands.

Because hands vary in size, there may be some initial difficulty in locating your exact pressure points, especially so if this is the first time you have attempted reflexology. A little practice will soon show where to find the right spot, principally by virtue of its tenderness, and you may even experience a physical sensation or sensitivity when you hit on the exact spot and start applying pressure to it.

Some reflexologists, too, maintain that they can locate the reflex point because it is often found sitting in a little depression into which the thumb tip slips and fits exactly as it glides over the skin. Experiment a little on your own palm and you will soon begin to recognize the differences from area to area.

When you have located the point, apply pressure to the spot by making slow, circular movements with the side of your thumbtip, but do take care to avoid jabbing yourself with your thumbnail. This gentle pressure is the reflexology massaging technique which relays a stimulating or analgesic message from the skin to its corresponding vital organ. And if, when you are applying pressure to a particular reflex point, you should feel any pain, it could be a clear indication that all is not well at the other end of the connection. The underlying principle of reflexology is that if there is any pain, by massaging the tender spot it is possible to rub the pain away.

Not only do a great number of conditions – from stress and tension, to organic disorders – respond to, and find relief through this type of massage, but its frequent use is claimed to stimulate the system, allowing its natural rejuvenating processes to take place.

Here is a selection of disorders which might benefit from daily massaging. The list has been simplified and kept necessarily brief. Many of the techniques can be carried out either when you feel any discomfort or as part of a daily routine to keep your system in tone. And, of course, because you are working on your hands, you can carry out your own therapy wherever you are.

STRESS AND TENSION
One aspect of a stessful life is that it tenses the abdominal muscles and thus impedes relaxation. You can obtain relief from nervous tension by massaging the solar plexus reflexes in both your hands. These are located centrally in the palms below your middle fingers.

MENTAL TIREDNESS
Brain fatigue, caused by too much mental or intellectual effort, as might occur during revision for exams, say, or following a relentless period of sustained mental activity, can be relieved by stimulating the brain reflexes located on the tips of your thumbs.

RESPIRATORY PROBLEMS
Breathing difficulties, bronchitis and asthma may respond to the stimulation of the lung reflexes, found across the top third of your palm beneath the two middle fingers. Massage of the adrenal reflex in both palms would especially help if you suffer with asthma.

DIGESTIVE DISORDERS
Acidity, indigestion, constipation and flatulence can bring severe discomfort. Massaging of the intestinal reflexes in both hands can

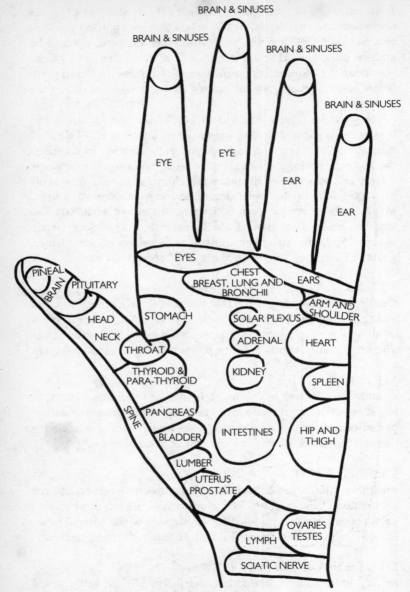

left hand Fig. 93

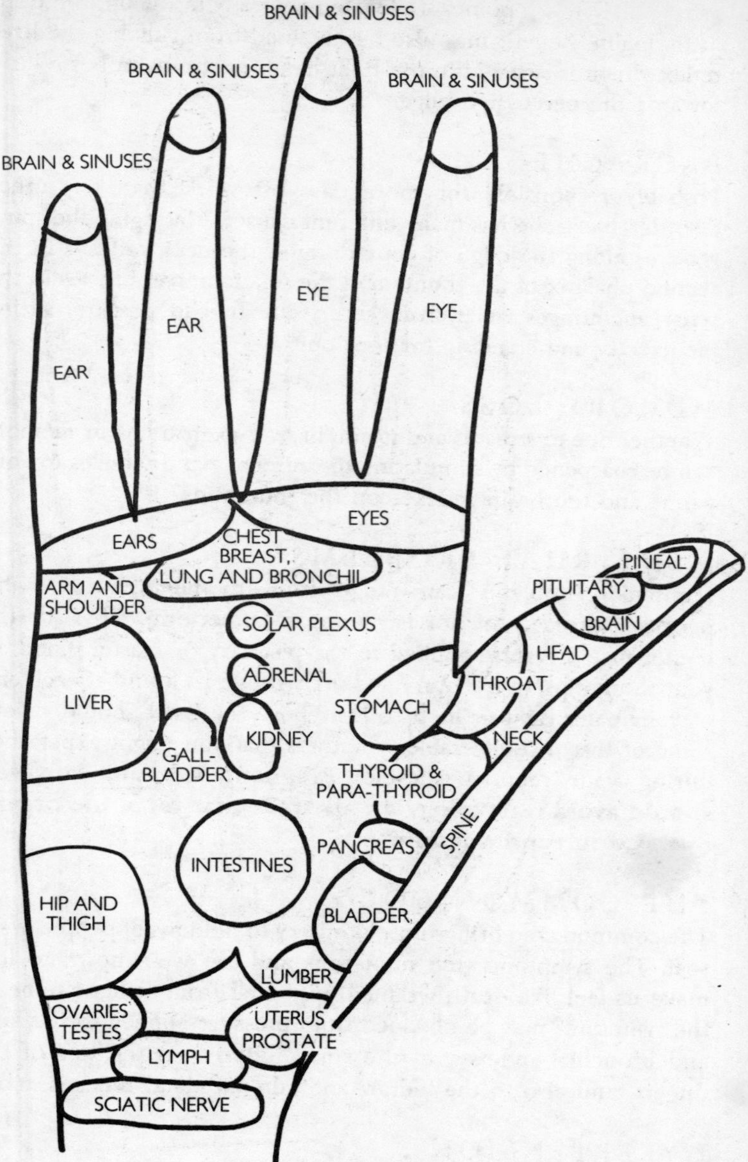

BRAIN & SINUSES

BRAIN & SINUSES

BRAIN & SINUSES

BRAIN & SINUSES

EYE

EYE

EAR

EAR

EAR

EYES

EARS

CHEST BREAST, LUNG AND BRONCHII

PINEAL

PITUITARY

BRAIN

ARM AND SHOULDER

SOLAR PLEXUS

HEAD

THROAT

ADRENAL

STOMACH

NECK

LIVER

KIDNEY

GALL-BLADDER

THYROID & PARA-THYROID

SPINE

PANCREAS

INTESTINES

BLADDER

HIP AND THIGH

LUMBER

OVARIES TESTES

UTERUS PROSTATE

LYMPH

SCIATIC NERVE

Fig. 93 right hand

bring relief. These points are located centrally in the bottom third of the palm. Benefit may also be obtained from rubbing the liver reflex which is situated in the right hand, centre palm but a little towards the percussion edge.

BACKACHE
Probably responsible for more days off work than any other disorder, backache has many different causes. Massaging the spine reflexes along the edge of your thumbs, the neck reflexes in the second phalanx of the thumb and the sciatic nerve reflexes in the wrist encourages relief from strain due to bad posture, sitting incorrectly and standing for too long.

MEMORY LOSS
Whether due to stresses and strain, or over-exertion, your memory can be sharpened by stimulating the adrenal gland reflexes in both palms and the brain reflexes on the thumbtips.

MENSTRUAL PROBLEMS
Menstrual problems can range from dysmenorrhea (painful periods), through menorrhagia (profuse periods), PMT to the menopause. Pressure applied to the pituitary or master gland on your thumbtips, to the ovary and uterus reflexes found at each end of your palm right at its base just above the wrist should relieve some of the uncomfortable symptoms that you might experience during your menstrual cycle. **Pregnant women, however, should avoid reflexology on all areas that relax the organs involved in reproduction.**

THE COMMON COLD
The common cold brings untold misery to millions of people every year. The symptoms, too numerous and too well-known to list, make us feel like death warmed up. Relief from at least some of the symptoms may be obtained from pressure applied to the lung and bronchial reflexes, to the sinus reflexes on the tips of the fingers, and also to the kidney and adrenal gland reflexes, too.

HYPERTENSION
High blood pressure is a serious condition which, if allowed to

continue uncontrolled, can result in serious heart problems and strokes. It is imperative, then, that a doctor be consulted if anyone suspects they suffer from this condition. However, there is a great deal of preventive work that reflexology can do to relieve some of the problems that cause the hypertension in the first place. Pressure applied to the following reflexes should help the symptoms: the heart, the kidneys and adrenals, the thyroid, the parathyroid, and the liver.

OBESITY

If you're on a diet and trying to lose weight, reflexology may be able to help. Encourage weight reduction by promoting your digestive system, stimulating the efficient elimination of wastes and thereby discouraging fluid retention. You can do this by applying pressure to the lymph gland reflexes, to the intestinal area, and to the kidney and liver reflexes. Carried out for a few minutes daily, this practice should make a good start in fighting the flab.

5

Massage for Body Toning

THE POWER OF TOUCH

Massage, as mentioned in the previous chapter, is a valuable therapeutic tool. Practised in every culture throughout the world, the healing power of touch has been recognized for thousands of years. And although scientifically it is still not possible to come up with a reason for the healing force of massage, its widespread use cannot be denied or ignored as a tool for soothing or stimulating the body's responses, for toning up the system, for the relief of pain and for encouraging the body's natural healing processes to take place.

In respect to the hand, massage has a dual appropriateness. Firstly, it is a therapy which involves manipulating the body of another person with our own hands and, secondly, many of the massage techniques can be applied directly to our own hands, and the benefits of this therapy will be directly relayed or transmitted to other parts of our systems.

Apart from reflexology, other techniques have been developed over the centuries, some using gentle pressure on the skin and soft tissues, whilst others, such as neuromuscular massage for example, apply weight and force in deep kneading or sawing movements intended to reach the deeper ligaments and tendons.

Certain types of massage are suited to specific parts of the body. Reflexology, for example, concentrates on feet, hands and ears. Shiatsu only works along the meridians that run down the body. Some manipulation can only be performed by a second person – reaching round to massage your own back without a partner or masseur to help is pretty nigh impossible. And then, of course, there are some therapies which should only be performed by professionally trained practitioners.

Massaging the hand, however, uniquely cuts through all these difficulties. Not only can it be carried out most satisfactorily by yourself, but the hand can be massaged unobtrusively even in a room full of people. Moreover, a combination of techniques can be used so as to benefit right across the spectrum of massage therapies. Reflexology, particularly suited to the hand, has been described in the previous chapter, but aromatherapy and acupressure can also be used, blending with them a variety of techniques such as effleurage and deep pressure massage.

Aromatherapy is especially delightful to use on the hands with its scented essences providing a twin function, both therapeutic and cosmetic. The essential oils used in aromatherapy are distilled from aromatic herbs and flowers and may be used to treat a variety of conditions. Neroli, for example, extracted from the flowers of the bitter orange tree, is used to treat nervous conditions. It contains tranquillizing properties which have been found to be of great benefit to the nervous system. Bergamot, on the other hand, is a tonic and makes a good antiseptic. Rosemary may be used as a stimulant and is especially beneficial in memory loss. Black pepper aids concentration whilst ylang ylang is an aphrodisiac.

And, of course, the oils may be mixed and blended to treat a wide spectrum of conditions according to the individual's need. But care must be taken before using aromatherapy oils because they are very concentrated and very potent and some have been known to set up adverse reactions. In addition, there are some oils which should not be used under certain conditions, such as in pregnancy, for example. And they should never be taken internally.

So, if you do decide to use these aromatic oils as part of your massaging routine, do a little homework first. Make sure the oils you want to use are recommended for promoting the very type of mental or physical state of well-being that you are seeking and that they don't clash with any medical condition you might be suffering from.

The massage technique mainly used on the hand for a general toning up of the system is effleurage. Here, a stroking movement is applied either with the whole hand or with the thumb, especially

so when massaging between the tendons. A light stroke has a
relaxing effect whilst more pressure will stimulate the circulatory
system and the deeper muscles and tissues beneath the surface.

Massage is always performed upwards, towards the heart, so that
even if working from the wrist down to the fingers, the pressure
movements are upswept in the direction of the arm and the
massaging hand allowed to trail lightly back down in a drawing
motion out through the fingers.

But whatever techniques are employed it must always be borne
in mind that massage is a powerful tool which can have surprising
effects even when just used on the hand.

THE BODY TONING HAND MASSAGE

You can massage your own hands by using one to work on the other.
Both the heel of your hand and the thumb can be used to apply
the pressure, and extended manipulation can be given to any tender
spots that are found. Although a lubricant is not absolutely
essential, it is very pleasant, nevertheless, if scented talcum powder
or aromatherapy oils are used. The choice of essence/s will
determine whether relaxing or stimulating effects are required.

None of the movements should be forced and especially not if
there is the slightest natural resistance or if injury or disease will
not permit.

1. Starting at the wrist, massage by pressing the tip of your thumb
   in light circular movements, horizontally across the wrist and
   over onto the back of the arm. This helps to loosen the muscles
   and ligaments at the wrist.
2. Press with the heel of one hand against the knuckles of the
   other so as to push the hand down perpendicularly to the wrist.
   Then, holding the arm outstretched and palm upwards, grasp
   the fingers and pull them downwards until you feel the tension
   at the wrist.
3. Repeat for the other hand.
4. With the palm of one hand resting on the backs of the fingers
   of the other, massage the back of the hand by pressing the
   thumbtip up between the tendons. These run from the digits
   up into the arm. Start from the webbing between the thumb
   and index, applying pressure upwards between the two

tendons and allowing the thumb action to trail lightly backwards on its return stroke.

5. In the same way, work between each of the four fingers, from the web applying pressure as the thumbtip is rubbed up between the tendons, and then allowed to trail back down again.

6. Repeat for the other hand.

7. Firmly pinch the four webs between each of your digits in turn for several seconds at a time. Toxins gather between your fingers and form little crystalline nodules in the web. By pinching and applying a circular motion between thumb and index, the nodules may be broken down and allowed to become eliminated by your body's natural cleansing mechanisms.

8. Repeat for the other hand.

9. Turning the hand around and starting at the base of the palm, apply pressure systematically with the thumb using small circular movements starting from the thumb edge and working horizontally across the palm to the percussion edge. Work right across the palm, section by section, until the whole palm has been covered. Any tender spots should be returned to periodically and worked on again for several seconds at a time.

10. Repeat for the other hand.

11. Starting with the tip of the thumb, apply the same massaging pressure in circular movements all the way down the digit, pinching and rubbing the joints en route.

12. Apply the same sequence of pressure massage to each of the fingers in turn. The major meridians feed out through the five digits, so this massaging will reach the acupressure points located in the fingers and thumbs.

13. Repeat the whole sequence on the digits of the other hand.

14. Interlace the fingers and stretch each hand against the other, feeling the pull and tension at the base of your fingers.

15. Shake your hands vigorously until they tingle.

Two further exercises, devised and pioneered by Dr Fitzgerald who brought reflexology to the West, may be added to the toning-up routine.

16. Grip a steel comb tightly in your fist with the teeth pressing into the base of your fingers. This will tone up your whole skeletal structure. Press the teeth of the comb firmly onto the very tips of your fingers for relief of aches and pains in your spine. If you have strong, long nails you have a ready-made substitute for the comb! Simply press the nails of one hand into the fingertips of the other for a few seconds. Swap over and do the other hand.

17. Apply clothes pegs to the tips of your fingers and leave for up to five minutes. Dr Fitzgerald's research found this of great benefit to the teeth, especially to help relieve the pain of toothache. Additionally, this exercise will stimulate the nervous system and, because the fingertips are endpoints of the meridians, it will also act as a tonic for the whole of the body, too.

And finally, whether the manipulation has been conducted by yourself or by another person, the hands should always be washed at the end of the massage routine.

Massage is not a miracle cure-all but a regular hand workout will benefit your whole nervous system, relaxing both mind and body. Additionally it will stimulate your blood circulation whilst also bringing relief to many existing conditions and preventing the onset of many others.

6

A–Z of Markings and Symptoms

Within our genetic make-up, we all of us have built-in weak links, tendencies and predispositions to particular disorders. Some of us are more susceptible than others to circulatory problems, for example, some to respiratory disorders, others to intestinal upsets. Some people may be physiologically weak whilst they are psychologically strong. Others are the other way round, able to withstand no end of physical hardship, but buckle under the strain immediately they're confronted with a mental or emotional crisis.

The information in this chapter is intended to make you aware of your strengths and weaknesses. It highlights your own personal susceptibilities according to the markings in your hand and mirrors both your mental and physical state of health. Taking note of your weak links and predispositions in this way not only gives you insight into the workings of your own body but also encourages you to take preventive action, to stave off any disorder you are particularly vulnerable to. It may also prompt you to seek medical advice well in advance of a condition flaring up into a full-blown clinical problem.

Throughout the book you have been urged to keep in mind two salient factors and they perhaps apply here more so than in any other chapter. Firstly, try not to diagnose from one single marking alone, or even from the hand alone. If you suspect that you have detected any serious condition, consult your doctor immediately. Secondly, do remember that lines can and do change so you may well have time to do something about any negative markings you come across. Change your attitude, your diet, your way of life and you will be surprised how quickly your hands will respond.

And always bear in mind that prevention is better than a cure!

THE HEALTH MAP

Although physicians thousands of years ago routinely and extensively consulted their patients' hands on matters of health, the modern, scientific study of health markings in the hand is still in its infancy. Today, patient medical research is being carried out and a good deal of information is now establishing links between certain diseases and specific lines and markings in the hand. Interestingly, some of the work is validating what those venerable physicians already knew such a long time ago. But equally, new and exciting findings and explanations are now being brought to light that it seems only a matter of time before medical hand analysis is accepted in the GP's surgery as an aid to diagnosis.

However, it is slow work and a good deal more needs to be done yet. There is a great deal that we know and far more that we still don't know. With many markings, we feel confident that an association with particular conditions exist, but other markings and their correlations are still conjectural. To add to the theories, I propose the following map. Here, known groups of markings and their associations with major organs and anatomical parts of the body have been charted into areas where they occur in the hand.

We have already established a link between markings on the fingertips corresponding to the nervous system in terms of the little horizontal worry lines. We suspect, too, a connection with the endocrine system, hormonal imbalances making their presence felt by vertical lines here.

Beneath the roots of the fingers, we believe, are markings which are associated with disorders of the eyes, the teeth, and the throat. Correlations with the cardiac and circulatory system, with the head, lungs and thorax are found in the area of the Heart and Head lines.

Centre palm sees markings that link with the organs of digestion and elimination, the liver, the kidneys, the gall-bladder.

Lower down, lines and markings across the thenar and hypothenar, or mounts of Venus and Luna, are connected with the organs of reproduction, the ovaries and testes.

Looking at this map, it is reassuring to note how many similarities there are between these health markings and the reflexology points as shown in Figure 93, pages 190-1.

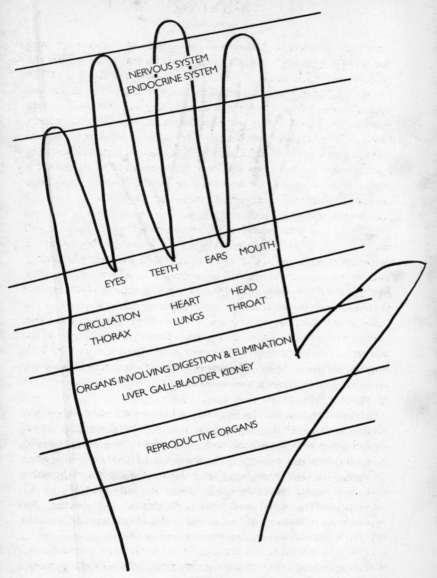

NERVOUS SYSTEM
ENDOCRINE SYSTEM

EYES   TEETH   EARS   MOUTH

HEAD

CIRCULATION   HEART   THROAT
              LUNGS

THORAX

ORGANS INVOLVING DIGESTION & ELIMINATION
LIVER, GALL-BLADDER, KIDNEY

REPRODUCTIVE ORGANS

Fig. 94

The A-Z

ACIDITY

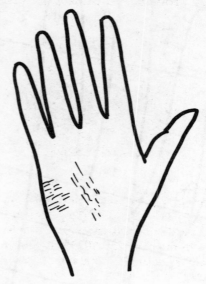

Fig. 95

Whether part of faulty digestion or a slow build-up in the system, signs of acidity may be represented by:

1. Flaring. These are fine lines like tongues of fire that run obliquely from the centre of the palm up towards the third and fourth fingers. This marking is particularly associated with a tendency to stomach or intestinal acidity, sometimes due to faulty diet and sometimes brought on by anxiety and stress.

2. Veiling on the percussion, that is, numerous fine superficial criss-crossing lines which cut across the ridge pattern in that section of the palm beneath the beginning of the Heart line. This marking is believed to represent a slow build-up of uric acid, which could trigger and aggravate certain rheumatic conditions.

• Of the tissue salts, Nat. Phos. and Nat. Mur. are the principal remedies used to combat the symptoms of acidity.

- Mint tea taken as an infusion may be of benefit. Both centaury and yarrow aid the digestive process.

See also **Kidney Problems, Rheumatic Diseases**

AIDS

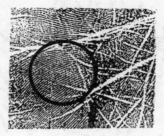

Fig. 96

Not enough research has as yet been carried out on sufferers of HIV syndrome to be able to put together a list of markings associated with the disease. Observations to date have recorded that the skin ridges in the palms of AIDS sufferers are fragmented, a symptom already associated with a vulnerable immune system.

- Mistletoe, though toxic in the wild, is said to strengthen the immune system when prepared herbally and may therefore be of some benefit here.

ALLERGIES
The major marking that points to physiological sensitivities to chemicals, drugs, etc. is the allergy line which is found lying horizontally across the hypothenar eminence, or mount of Luna (see Figure 97, overleaf). Unfortunately, whilst the presence of the line does point to a general sensitivity to allergens, it does not distinguish the allergens to which the individual may be allergic.

- Check for stress markings which may also be present in the hand as some conditions are stress-related.
- Keeping records of diet and contact with chemicals together with adverse reactions may isolate particular allergens.
- Vitamin C and garlic may be of benefit.

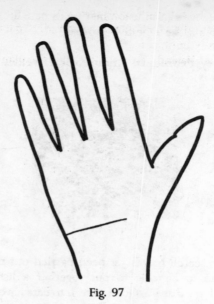

Fig. 97

ANAEMIA

1. A pale or even white skin on the hands is a first clue to anaemia.
2. When fingers are flexed backwards, the lines look pale or even run to white. Dryness and exposure to chemicals may equally be responsible for this, so environmental factors must be taken into consideration first. Often the lines can look pale after menstruation, when a good deal of iron has been lost in the menstrual flow.

    If feeling tired, or drained, or washed out following a period, and you suspect a tendency to anaemia, try to avoid reaching for the iron pills (unless, of course, medically prescribed) as these can upset your stomach and intestines. Consider, instead, boosting the blood by natural means or by supplementation as listed below.

- Iron-rich foods including green-leaf vegetables, liver, molasses, fish and shellfish, raisins and nuts.
- Vitamin B complex, particularly B12.

- Vitamin C to aid iron absorption.
- Calc. Phos. and Ferr. Phos. are the two principal tissue salts used in anaemic conditions.
- Herbally, alfalfa and nettle are amongst the plants listed for this condition.

ANXIETY - *See* **Nervous Disorders**

ARTHRITIS - *See* **Rheumatic Diseases**

ASTHMA - *See* **Respiratory Problems**

BACKACHE

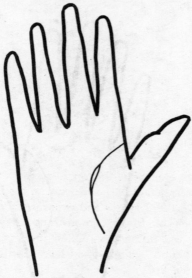

Fig. 98

Responsible for more days off work than any other ailment, backache is a complex problem as it can be a symptom of a variety of diseases, whether organic, mechanical or psychological. Some conditions may be due to injury, to general wear and tear, some to pain referred from other areas altogther and some may be congenital in origin.

The main indication of back or spinal trouble is seen in an island which occurs half-way down the Life line.

Of help in some cases may be the following vitamins and minerals:

- B complex, Vitamin C and calcium.
- Of the tissue salts recommended, Ferr. Phos. works on strains and sprains as well as on muscle stiffness high in the neck. Combination G, comprising Calc. Fluor., Calc. Phos., Kali Phos. and Nat. Mur., is used in the treatment of backache and lumbago.

BRONCHITIS – *See* **Respiratory Problems**

CANCER

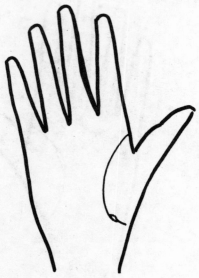

Fig. 99

Not enough reliable data exists to link markings categorically with the different types of cancers. Some signs which are suspected of being associated with the disease are listed below although many possessing the markings have never been found to develop cancer at all. Conversely, there are those individuals who have developed the disease whilst not showing any of these markings. Tentative, but by no means fool-proof, suggestions include:

1. Broken ridge lines.
2. A clear, well-formed island low down in the Life line.
3. Little yellowish, wart-like clusters of skin, similar to tiny calluses, which may occur on either the thenar or hypothenar eminences, that is, the Venus or Luna mounts. Some practitioners have suggested that a similar marking may occur running down the outside edge of the thumb towards the wrist.

CARDIO-VASCULAR PROBLEMS - *See* **Heart and Circulatory Problems**

DENTAL PROBLEMS

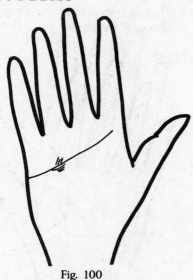

Fig. 100

Whether due to poor diet or to inherited orthodontal problems, tooth decay or other associated disorders affecting the teeth may be represented by:

1. Tiny oblique lines lying just over the Heart line directly below the webbing between the ring and little fingers. These should not be confused with the Medical Stigmata, also composed of oblique lines and also found around the same location. The

difference is that the marking of the Medical Stigmata is much larger and usually composed of a group of three lines, often crossed by a fourth horizontal one.

2. A series of little lines forming a ladder below the Heart line directly beneath the ring and little finger suggests a calcium deficiency which could well affect the teeth and gums.

- Calcium is essential for building healthy teeth.
- Calc. Phos. and Calc. Fluor. are recommended for decay and for the promotion of good enamel. Combination R, comprising Calc. Fluor., Calc. Phos., Ferr. Phos., Mag. Phos. and Silica, contains all the tissue salts required in the formation of good teeth, in the relief of troublesome teething, to ease toothache and other problems of dentition.

DEPRESSION

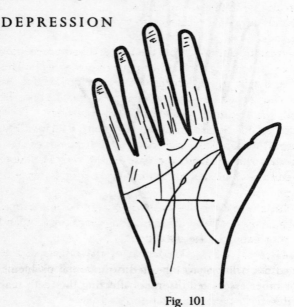

Fig. 101

Depression is one of those umbrella terms which covers a multitude of disorders from serious mental disease to simply feeling down or blue or melancholic. Though it is quite natural to go through periods of ups and downs, of feeling downright miserable on hearing bad news, say, or because of poor living conditions or even because the weather is uncongenial, true depression is a medical condition which may, in some people, last for a considerable period of time and severely affect their lives and their work.

Causes and actual periods of depression may be denoted in the hand by a variety of markings:

1. Islands in the Head line usually suggest times of worry and anxiety which may well spark off a period of depression.
2. Perhaps one of the best indications of a bout of depression is seen by a dip in the Head line from the apex of which shoots out a tiny downswept branch.
3. A markedly curved Head line flowing deep into the Hypothenar or Mount of Luna suggests an overactive mentality where the imagination can sometimes run wild.
4. The 'full hand' reveals a tendency to hypersensitivity and to neurotic moods.
5. A heavy trauma line cutting across the Life line and proceeding further up to cut through the other major lines as well. This represents a major upset which could potentially lead to depression. The deeper, the stronger and the longer the line, the more impact the traumatic event has upon its owner.
6. An over-developed Saturn mount is often a sign of a predisposition to depression, melancholia and moodiness.
7. Deep lines that run up from the base of the fingers denote chronic tiredness which can all too often bring on a sense of despondency.
8. Horizontal lines across the tips of the fingers indicate personal problems which may confirm other markings of depression and point to a root cause of the condition.
9. Vertical lines across the top phalanges of the fingers denote hormonal activity which may trigger serious mood swings.

Suggested strategies to fight the condition include:

• Vitamin C.
• Amino acid complex may be helpful.
• Magnesium and B6 as a deficiency may be a contributing factor in depression.

- Exposure to bright light has been found to be of benefit in the condition known as SAD syndrome (Seasonal Affective Disorder).
- Californian poppy for its sedative properties, ginseng as a tonic and for its stimulant action. A herbal infusion of valerian is recommended for hysteria, for nervous exhaustion and agitation of all kinds. Borage, or its flowers, taken as an infusion is a cheerful pick-me-up.
- Kali. Phos., Calc. Phos. and Nat. Mur. to dispel gloom and lift depression.

DIGESTIVE PROBLEMS

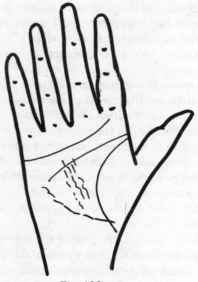

Fig. 102

This category includes a variety of disorders of the alimentary canal, the gut and intestines.

Markings which highlight these problems include:

1. Fine flaring lines rising obliquely from the centre of the palm up towards the ring finger suggests the individual is prone to intestinal overactivity.

2. Other intestinal problems may be represented by a Luna mount which is heavily marked by lines.
3. Flabbiness of the basal phalanx of the index finger can denote a tendency to dyspepsia, mainly due to faulty nutrition.
4. Disorders of the gall-bladder may be indicated by a triangular or diamond-shaped group of lines attached to the Life line, some two-thirds of the way down the palm.
5. A fragmented health line may signify gastric and intestinal disorders.

- Nat. Phos. is a tissue salt that is reputed to fight against acidity. Silica, also recommended for this condition, is more helpful in eliminating chronic acidity but is a very slow worker.
- A vast range of herbal teas and preparations exist to aid digestion: peppermint for indigestion and for easing nausea and stomach pain; thyme and balm mint for stomach cramps and diarrhoea; fennel for colic; dandelion as a blood purifier; ginger and pineapple for dyspepsia, for difficulty in digesting food, for nausea and for treating lack of appetite.
- Two major groups of tissue salts are held in high regard in easing gastric disorders. Combination C, consisting of Mag. Phos., Nat. Phos., Nat. Sulph. and Silica, for all conditions involving acidity, heartburn and indigestion. Combination S, comprising Kali. Mur., Nat. Phos. and Nat. Sulph., for treating acute stomach upsets, nausea and biliousness.

EYES

1. A large island in the Heart line beneath the ring finger is a classic symptom said to denote a tendency to ophthalmic problems. However, an island here may also represent heart or circulatory problems, so some confusion may occur.
2. Another marking which may suggest problems with vision is an island in the Head line beneath the mount of Apollo.
3. Some practitioners claim that a circular or semi-circular marking either above the Heart line beneath the ring finger, or attached to the inside edge of the Life line is a symptom of a susceptibility to cataracts.

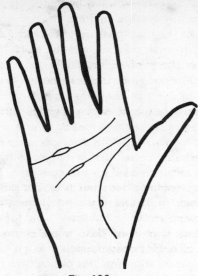

Fig. 103

- Vitamin A is essential for healthy eyes.
- Eyebright, either taken internally as an infusion or made up into a lotion or as a compress and applied to the eyes, is a traditional remedy in the treatment of weak or diseased eyes. The herb is also reputed to boost sight.
- Carrot and bilberry capsules are recommended for night blindness.
- Silica for the treatment of sties; Kali. Phos. for weakness; Nat. Mur. for watery eyes; Ferr. Phos. for pain, inflammation and redness.

FEVER

1. People prone to feverish conditions tend to possess a full mount of Apollo.
2. High fever often leaves a horizontal groove across all the nails. Because on average a nail takes roughly six months to grow from the cuticle to the top of the quick (that is, the pink living part of the nail), it is possible to date when the illness took place.

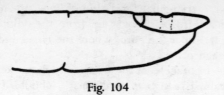

Fig. 104

Close to the base would suggest a recent onslaught, across the middle implies about three months previously, and nearer the top would indicate that the illness occurred some five to six months earlier.

- Borage has a cooling action and as such is used in the treatment of fevers. Eucalyptus, too, may help in cases where the condition is intermittent.
- Of the tissue salts, Ferr. Phos. is the primary remedy in the treatment of feverish conditions.

GYNAECOLOGICAL DISORDERS

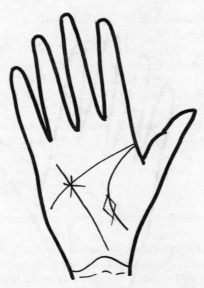

Fig. 105

1. A diamond or triangular formation of lines attached to the Life line about a third of the way up from the palm.
2. A star formation at the point where the Head and Health lines intersect each other.
3. A rascette - or bracelet at the wrist - which markedly humps up into the palm is a sign of problems in childbirth.

- Sage is a key herb recommended for painful and irregular menstruation, for PMT and general menopausal problems; hops and alfalfa for hormonal regulation; motherwort and camomile for their soothing properties; shepherd's purse against internal haemorrhaging, especially of the uterus.
- Because this category covers a wide range of disorders, there is an equally wide variety of biochemic remedies to suit. Combination N, however, comprising Calc. Phos., Kali. Mur., Kali. Phos. and Mag. Phos., are recommended for painful periods and other allied gynaecological problems.

See also **Reproductive System Disorders**

HEADACHES AND MIGRAINE

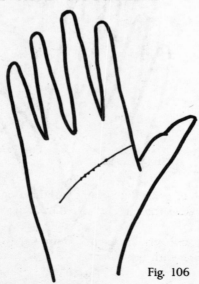

Fig. 106

A tendency to headaches and particularly to migraine may be detected by tiny indentations in the Head line. Often these are grouped together, highlighting periods when the attacks are more concentrated.

- Calcium is said to be of benefit.
- Though an old herbal remedy, feverfew is now gaining recognition in orthodox medical circles as a potent cure for migraine.
- Of the tissue salts, Combination F is recommended for headaches and migraine. Combined in this formulation are Kali. Phos., Mag. Phos., Nat. Mur. and Silica.

HEARING PROBLEMS

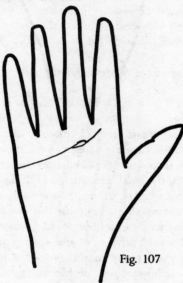

Fig. 107

A classic sign of general problems with hearing is an island in the Heart line below the middle, or Saturn, finger.

- Kali. Mur. and Ferr. Phos. are the two key tissue salts of benefit in problems with the ears.

HEART AND CIRCULATORY PROBLEMS

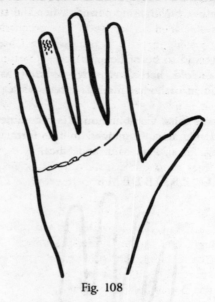

Fig. 108

Problems of the heart and circulation are many and varied. Conditions included in this category of illnesses range from high blood pressure, through angina and arteriosclerosis, to coronary or heart disease. Of the small percentage of these disorders which are genetic or congenital in origin, abnormalities in the skin ridge patterns may throw some light on the conditions. The greater majority are due to diet, to lifestyle, to environmental factors and to the general wear and tear of the ageing process.

There are a good many markings in the hand which show a tendency to cardio-vascular problems and, though individuals possessing one or even two of these features need not necessarily develop a clinical condition, if any problems are suspected, however, a physician should be consulted at the earliest opportunity.

Markings include:

1. Short, often triangular or shell-shaped nails are a sign of a susceptibility to hypertension, or high blood pressure.

2. Of the skin ridge-patterns, the arched fingerprints are perhaps more associated with a predisposition to heart complaints than other patterns. More significant is an axial triradius pattern which is displaced higher up on the percussion towards the Heart line. This marking is discussed in Chapter 2.

3. The structure and condition of the Heart line reflects the workings of the heart and the circulation. Features which may here point to weaknesses of the cardio-vascular system include: a line that is chained along a large proportion of its course; a single weak thin line with no feathering, islanding or chained effects at its beginning where it enters the palm at the percussion edge; a marked break in the Heart line; a cluster of cross lines formed into a star that sits over the line; a single large blue island in the line below either the ring or little fingers.

4. Bulbous or clubbed fingertips.

5. Cyanosis, or blue discolouration of the nails and skin.

6. The Simian line suggests the possibility of a genetic or congenital predisposition to heart or circulatory problems.

7. A star formation sitting over the Head line may, in some cases, suggest the possibility of a stroke.

8. A heavily lined tip on the ring finger is believed to be associated with high blood pressure. The lines in this case are vertical not horizontal ones.

9. Very red hands or unnaturally red lines are associated with high blood pressure.

10. Studies have shown that in some cases nodules, or little hard lumps, may develop around the Heart line beneath the ring finger either immediately prior to, or following a heart attack.

11. Cold hands and fingers point to poor circulation.

12. Horizontal white lines across the nails, which are known as Mee's lines, are associated with heart disease.

Diet – especially cutting out salt and reducing alcohol intake – exercise and weight reduction and, of course, giving up smoking, are considered essential in maintaining good circulation and a healthy heart. Dietary advice from recent research into heart disease suggests that regular intake of the following is not only beneficial to the action of the heart but helps to prevent disease:

- Garlic tablets daily.
- Oily fish.
- GLA, particularly concentrated in oil of evening primrose.
- Reduction of saturated fats and an increase of mono- or polyunsaturated fats.
- Because the conditions under this category are so varied, herbal preparations should be taken on advice as each will be specific to particular complaints. Garlic is recommended for lowering high blood pressure, whereas broom is said to increase pressure. Bamboo gum is held to be of value in atherosclerosis, or hardening of the arteries. Gugulon is believed to lower cholesterol; ginkgo to boost circulation.
- Amongst the tissue salts recommended to stimulate the circulation are: Kali. Phos., Calc. Phos. and Calc. Fluor.

HERNIA

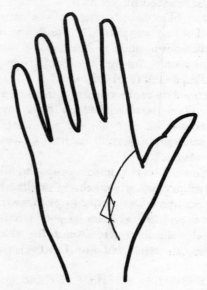

Fig. 109

A tendency to hernia may be marked by a diamond or triangular-shaped formation of lines attached to the Life line about two-thirds of the way down the palm.

HERPES SIMPLEX

A viral condition believed to be aggravated by stress, Herpes Simplex begins with irritation in isolated spots on, or between, the fingers and sometimes on the palm. The affected area of skin reddens and little watery vesicles subsequently develop.

HYPERTENSION or HIGH BLOOD PRESSURE

See **Heart and Circulatory Problems**

HYPER- AND HYPOTHYROIDISM

See **Thyroid Imbalance**

INDIGESTION

See **Digestive Problems**

INSOMNIA

See **Sleep Disorders**

LIVER DYSFUNCTION

Problems with the liver may produce the following symptoms:

1. Yellowish tinge to the skin on the hands, and a yellow discolouration of the nails.
2. A broken Health line.

- Fumitory stimulates the secretion of bile; liverwort purifies the blood; centaury relieves pain in the liver and the spleen; dandelion tones up a sluggish liver.
- Nat. Sulph. is recommended in disorders of the liver and gall-bladder and Kali. Sulph. in aiding the sluggish action of the liver.

MEMORY LOSS

Many conditions may impair the memory, the most common of which is the slow erosion that comes with age. Forgetfulness may occur at any time in life, particularly so when the individual is going through an especially busy period. But clinical memory loss, whether caused by injury or diseases of the brain or of the nervous

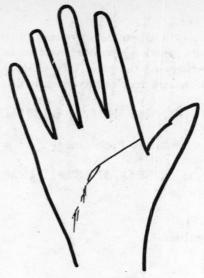

Fig. 110

system, such as dementia, for example may be registered in the hand by a thinning and fraying of the Head line towards its end. In some cases, the line may visibly wilt downwards towards the Luna mount and may be chained, feathered or fragmented.

- Minerals and tissue salts that are said to tone the memory include zinc, Calc. Fluor. and Silica.
- Herbal preparations to improve memory and concentration include ginseng, schisandra and pollen capsules. The latter is especially recommended for the elderly.

MENSTRUAL PROBLEMS
See **Reproductive System Disorders**

NERVOUS DISORDERS
A large catch-all category that includes all manner of nervous upsets, agitation, anxiety and nervousness. Highly-strung individuals prone to a variety of conditions affecting the nervous system

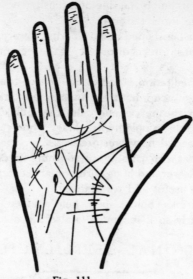

Fig. 111

including neurosis, nervous tension and nervous anxiety will be
revealed by the following features:

1. The 'full hand'. This term applies to a hand that is literally
   covered in fine lines that criss-cross the whole palm rather like
   a spider's web.
2. A lean oblong-shaped palm with long, lean fingers accompanied
   by a weak-looking thumb.
3. An over-developed Mercury mount which is much marked and
   lined.
4. A bulge high on the percussion directly beneath the little finger
   is always a tell-tale sign of an overactive and fretful type of
   mentality.
5. A long curved Head line that slopes deeply into the mount of
   Luna denotes a heightened imagination and a temperament
   which is perhaps more prone to neurosis.
6. A series of fine horizontal lines that cut across the Life line are
   a sign of an anxious personality.

7. The Simian line is the sign of intensity and as such is associated with deep inner tension.
8. Wedge or fan-shaped nails, tapering towards the base, highlight a predisposition to disorders of the nervous system.

- Yoga, meditation, relaxation, deep-breathing techniques, reflexology, acupuncture, aromatherapy may all help to soothe and relax the nerves and calm the individual.
- Of the salt supplements, Mag. Phos. and Kali. Phos are recommended nerve restoratives.
- Herbal teas with calming and soothing effects include camomile.
- Passion flower and hops both contain sedative properties which are both useful and restorative.
- Milky drinks before bed help induce relaxed sleep and particularly so if insomnia is also a problem.

NUTRITIONAL DEFICIENCIES

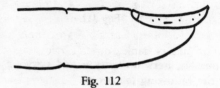

Fig. 112

Signs of nutritional deficiencies are mainly concentrated in the nails. The reason for this lies in the fact that nail production is a continuous process and is particularly sensitive to changes in the constituents and supply of blood. Any hiccups or interruptions, such as a sudden crash diet for example, will affect production and find an immediate response in the actual fabric and construction of the nail.

Sudden or acute nutritional deficiencies are usually denoted by a single mark on each nail which eventually grows out. More chronic conditions, however, may actually affect the very shape and construction of the nail itself.

Because it is known that nails take on average six months to grow, any marking in the nail can be timed, thus giving a pretty clear idea of when the illness or incident took place. A marking low down on the nail suggests a recent occurrence, higher up implies some three months previously and towards the top would denote roughly six months earlier.

Signs of nutritional deficiencies in the hand include:

1. Spoon- or concave-shaped nails.
2. White specks in the nails.
3. Horizontal grooves across the nails.
4. Very soft nails, especially ones that split or break easily.
5. Lines in the palm that run pale when the fingers are flexed back.
6. Chronic or long-term deficiency will lead to a break-down of the skin ridges.

• It is said that serious nutritional deficiencies are unlikely to occur in the West where the majority of people can afford to eat a balanced diet. Yet deformities and markings in the nails described here are commonly seen by the average hand analyst, which suggests that nutritional deficiencies are rife. It is now widely accepted that modern processing techniques and agricultural practices of crop-spraying strip out of our foodstuffs the vitamins and minerals which are so essential for optimum health. Or perhaps it is that our dietary habits, our lifestyles, our constant urge to monitor our intake in order to lose weight, in fact deprives us of the basic nutrients we require to keep healthy. Certainly, medical researchers would agree that many Western diseases, such as cancer, heart and circulation problems, are diet-related.

And it is because of this that many turn to vitamin and mineral supplementation to make up the deficit. However, because of their interrelated action, vitamins and minerals should not be taken in isolation, because too much of one can seriously deplete another and very soon a serious imbalance will be set up. So for best effect a multi-vitamin and mineral tablet is perhaps the safest way to boost nutrition and it is strongly recommended not to exceed the stated dose.

See also **Vitamin and Mineral Deficiencies**

OBESITY

Signs of either a tendency to put on weight easily or of overweightness itself may be shown by the following features:

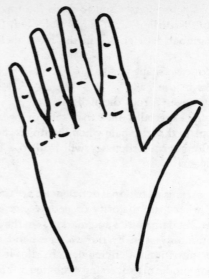

Fig. 113

1. Soft, plump basal phalanges on all the fingers is a sign of a sensual, self-indulgent and often indolent individual. People with these fingers are invariably overweight.
2. If little fat pads are present on the basal phalanges on the backs of the fingers, the weight problem is more long-term and has probably been building up since childhood. Consequently, it will be more difficult to shift the excess weight.

- Will-power, exercise and a carefully calorie-controlled diet are fundamentally the best ways of losing weight. Crash diets are not recommended as these can set up all sorts of nutritional deficiencies and imbalances in the system. Those who are very overweight should check with their doctors first before undertaking any weight-loss programmes.
- Some herbalists maintain that preparations do exist which aid weight-loss and name green tea (Camelia Thea), guarana and bean husk among them. Preparations from the pineapple plant are reputed to act against cellulitis.

REPRODUCTIVE SYSTEM DISORDERS

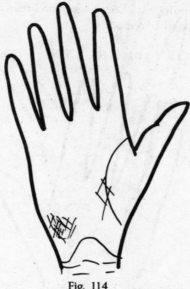

Fig. 114

The area in the hand representing the reproductive organs is located at the base of the palm just above the wrist. Markings that draw attention to possible problems involving these organs include:

1. A fine tracery of lines that cover the base of the hypothenar, or mount of Luna.
2. A pattern of lines that form themselves into either a diamond or a triangular shape attached to the Life line about two-thirds of the way down its course.
3. The top rascette arching steeply up into the base of the palm may imply a tendency to problems during childbirth.

- Calcium sulphate may benefit in cases of impotency.
- Check sodium/potassium imbalance marked by fine chaining of Head and Heart line. An imbalance may in part contribute to PMT.

- Oil of evening primrose is claimed to have some effect on regularizing the menstrual cycle.

See also **Gynaecological Disorders** for further information on biochemic and herbal remedies.

RESPIRATORY PROBLEMS

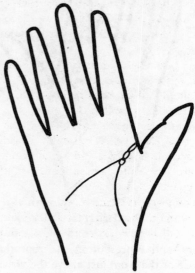

Fig. 115

A large category of disorders comprising sore throats, bronchitis, pneumonia, tuberculosis and lung disease. Signs representing either a predisposition or marking actual problems include:

1. A predisposition to respiratory problems may be registered by islands at the beginning of the Head line.
2. The nails curve around the tip of the finger. The process of curving appears to follow a set pattern, begining with the nail on the left index finger followed by the right, the left middle finger, then the right one, and subsequently the rest of the digits.
3. More severe cases are marked by the humped nail. Here the nail

rises up from the cuticle and, observed from the side, resembles a humped bridge as it arches from base to tip.

4. With some types of serious respiratory conditions the fingertips may swell and distort and take on a 'clubbed' appearance which is characteristic of advanced lung disease. Clubbed fingertips may also occur with heart disease and severe problems of the circulatory system.

5. Also in advanced cases, cynanosis, or a blue colour, may tinge the nails as well as the skin. The blue discolouration is also associated with certain cardio-vascular problems.

- Of the tissue salts, Kali. Mur. is said to be of benefit with congestion and sore throats. Preparation Q, a combination of Ferr. Phos., Kali. Mur., Kali. Phos. and Nat. Mur., is recommended for catarrh and sinus problems.

- Infusions made with thyme and elecampane are held to be effective in that they relax muscular spasms and have an expectorant action. Coltsfoot and white horehound made into herbal teas are especially recommended in the treatment of coughs and colds.

- Ephedra (which gives its name to ephedrine, a drug prescribed for problems with the respiratory tract) and plantain are also used for asthmatic and bronchitic conditions and allied problems.

RHEUMATIC DISEASES

The general characteristic of rheumatic disorders is that of inflammation of the joints. Included in this class of diseases is not only rheumatism itself, but also gout, osteoarthrosis and rheumatoid arthritis. The painful inflammation and progressive degeneration of these diseases, especially so in rheumatoid arthritis, can cause serious distortion of the joints, fingers and knuckles.

1. One of the first indications of rheumatism is swollen joints and in the more crippling form of rheumatoid arthritis, the knuckles may be mis-shapen and the fingers badly distorted.

2. An early sign of a predisposition to rheumatism in general may be seen by veiling on the percussion. This is a term used to describe a dense cluster of fine lines that cut through the skin ridge-pattern. When they occur on the percussion edge just

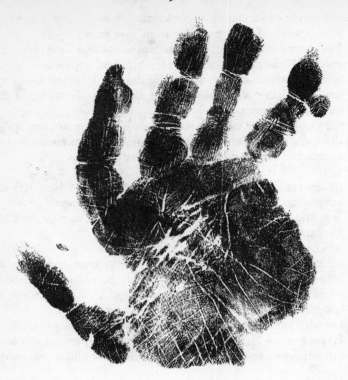

Fig. 116

below the Heart line they suggest a build-up of acidity which
may be implicated in the triggering and aggravation of rheumatic
conditions.

3. Heavy horizontal ridging of the nails is associated with this
   disease.

4. Very full basal phalanges show that the diet is faulty and if the
   base of the index finger is particularly large, it may well be
   illustrating a predisposition to rheumatic problems. If all basal
   phalanges are podgy in this way, perhaps a change of diet might
   help to stave off the development of the disease.

5. A large Luna mount that is heavily marked with lines may well
   point to a susceptibility to rheumatic problems.

Supplements and dietary suggestions include:

- Silica and Nat. Phos. amongst the tissue salts.
- Cod liver oil.
- Vitamin C.
- A large range of herbal preparations containing anti-inflammatory properties exist and are therefore of great benefit in these conditions. Devil's claw and Bamboo gum both help to relieve the pain in the joints and restore some mobility.

SLEEP DISORDERS

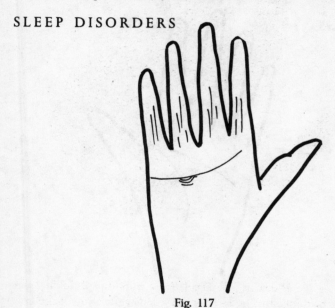

Fig. 117

A tendency to insomnia and broken sleep patterns may be registered in the following ways:

1. A tiny ladder-like series of lines beneath the Heart line roughly below the ring finger. When present, not only is the marking highlighting that the sleep pattern is disturbed, but by implication suggests that the nervous system is under stress, too.
2. Vertical lines that travel up the two basal phalanges of the fingers.

- The marking may be caused by a deficiency of calcium, or by a calcium/magnesium imbalance.
- Hot milky drinks before bed often have a calming and restful effect and thereby aid relaxed sleep.
- Camomile tea is reputed to be a great soother and is therefore of benefit before bedtime.
- Kali. Phos. may be of benefit if nervousness or excitability leads to restless sleep; Nat. Sulph. and Nat. Mur. are useful when sleep is not refreshing.

STRESS

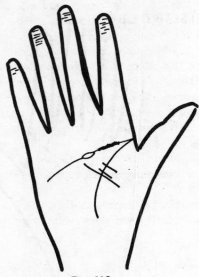

Fig. 118

Stress is the modern disease brought on by a variety of environmental pressures and everyday living conditions. It is now considered that stress is at the root cause of many of our ills, triggering numerous diseases from the common cold to cancer.

1. Horizontal lines across the fingertips are some of the first indicators of stress. As each digit governs a specific aspect of our lives, a greater concentration of these 'white lines', as they are called, on any particular finger will point to the underlying

cause of the problem. These stress markings and finger associations are dealt with in Chapter 3.

2. A single island in the Head line below the middle finger is a classic sign that its owner cannot cope with high pressure and should therefore steer clear of mentally taxing or over-demanding situations.

3. A fuzzy or 'woolly' section of the Head line denotes a period when greater mental demands are put on the individual and warns, therefore, of a time of stress. The beginning, duration and end of this period can be timed on the line.

4. Long-term or chronic stress can damage the actual skin ridges, causing them to break up. The disjointed patterning is easier to pick up on a print rather than with the naked eye on a living hand. When the ridges start to break down in this way, it is a sign that the whole constitution has been weakened and a warning that now the body is more vulnerable to disease. When the constitution is strengthened again, the ridges fairly rapidly re-knit themselves back into their normal long continuous lines.

- Kali. Phos. is the key tissue salt which helps to relax the system. Mag. Phos. relaxes tense nerves, especially if the stress produces headaches.
- Camomile tea is a great nerve soother, as are catmint and lemon balm. Capsules made from the passion flower plant ease anxiety and stress.

See also **Nervous Disorders**

STROKE
Possible signs that may denote a tendency to stroke include:

1. A star formation on the Head line.
2. Two long branches shooting out of the Heart line and descending down into the mount of Luna.
3. A predominant mount of Jupiter always suggests a large appetite, a penchant for rich foods and strong drink. Individuals who pursue this kind of high living are often apoplectic types and as such predisposed to stroke.

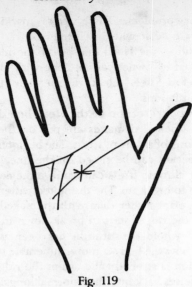

Fig. 119

- Silica, though slow-acting, is reputed to act on the arterial walls, making them stronger and more elastic.
- Recent research has found Vitamin E, or tocopherol, of value in maintaining healthy circulation and regulating blood pressure. But care *must* be taken by sufferers with hypertension when they first start taking this vitamin for it can have marked adverse effects if taken suddenly in too high a dosage. For these people, it is recommended that they begin with a very low dosage at first, no more that 100iu daily and very, very slowly build up to no more than 400iu.

See also **Heart and Circulatory Problems**

SURGERY
Presence of a marking need not imply that surgery is inevitable, merely that there is a susceptibility to a condition which may necessitate surgical intervention.

1. Certain conditions that may require an internal operation are sometimes denoted by a group of lines that form themselves into

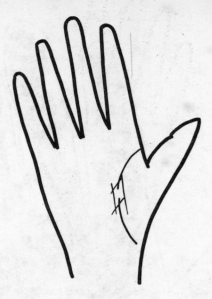

Fig. 120

either a diamond or a triangular pattern attached to the Life line about two-thirds of the way down the palm. This pattern is found in many hands and may correlate to a variety of different disorders ranging from digestive problems involving the gall-bladder, diseases of the female reproductive organs which may require a hysterectomy, hiatus hernia and urological disorders in men.

2. A clean break in the Life line. If one hand only shows the break, there may be mitigating markings which offset any need for surgery. A square over the break, for example, or a secondary inner line overlapping the break act as protection markings. If both hands show the same break at the same point in time the chances that there will be a need for surgery will be that much more likely – though, of course, still not inevitable!

TEETH
See **Dental Problems**

THYROID IMBALANCE

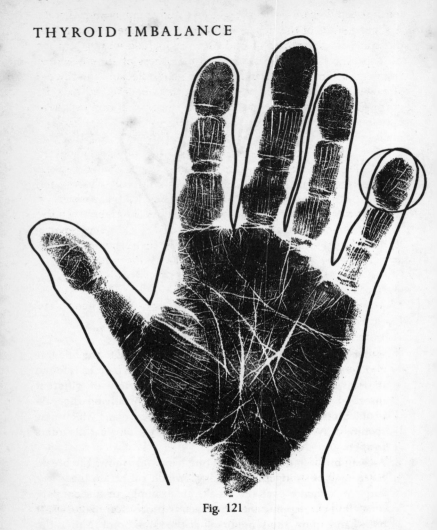

Fig. 121

Problems with the thyroid occur when the gland malfunctions and becomes either overactive, and thus produces too much thyroxine, or underactive and produces too little of the hormone. Both conditions have serious implications on growth and metabolism. Symptoms of overactivity include hyperactive behaviour, nervous tension, rapid heart action, weight loss, and damp, clammy hands. A slight tremor of the fingers also occurs when the arms are held outstretched. Symptoms of underactivity include weight gain for no apparent reason, general lethargy, slowness of speech and of response, aching muscles and cold, dry hands. Because the thyroid gland is part of the endocrine system, it is believed to have its correspondence on the tip of the little finger and markings here have been observed in the hands of those who suffer from a malfunction of the gland.

The most salient markings associated with an imbalance are vertical lines that run up the tip of the little finger. Sometimes, the lines are so numerous and so dense that they actually obscure the fingerprint. These markings, whilst showing a predisposition to thyroid problems, do not, or so we believe, distinguish between the over- or under-active condition but do, nevertheless suggest that the gland may be stressed. But there are further symptoms which are specifically associated with either one or the other:

Overactive or Hyperthyroidism:
1. A fine tremor of the fingers occurs when the hands are outstretched.
2. A smooth skin with a satin sheen to it.
3. Nails with markedly heavy horizontal ridging.
4. Very large moons in the nails.
5. Damp, clammy hands.

Underactive or Hypothyroidism:
1. Dry, cold, rough hands.
2. Concave or 'spoon' nails.
3. Nails may lack all moons.
4. Brittle nails that split or break easily.

- Iodine in kelp or seaweed tablets, Calc. Iodide and magnesium are said to be of value in thryroid disorders.

TIREDNESS
Tiredness may show up in the hand in a variety of ways:

1. Deep lines that run vertically up the two basal phalanges of the

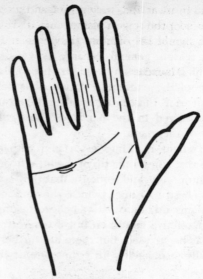

Fig. 122

fingers are a sign of tiredness.
2. A ladder-like series of little lines leading up to the Heart line beneath the ring finger show that the sleep pattern is disturbed.
3. Lines that run white when the fingers are flexed back show a lack of iron. This is a classic sign of iron-deficiency anaemia which is a very common nutrient deficiency. This feature often occurs after menstruation, especially so if the periods are heavy.

- Of the salt supplements, Mag. Phos., Ferr. Phos. and Kali. Phos. may help combat tiredness.
- When iron deficiency is suspected it is best to right the problem by eating foods rich in iron rather than by self-prescribing iron supplements such as ferrous sulphate, for example, which can be harsh on the digestion and may even cause constipation. Iron-rich foods include green vegetables such as spinach, liver, shellfish, raisins and molasses.
- Both calcium and Vitamin C help the absorption of iron.
- Vegans are especially prone to iron deficiency because their diet

excludes both meat and dairy products. Increasing their intake of soya-based products, molasses, dried fruit and green leaf vegetables should help restore the balance.

See also **Sleep Disorders**

URINARY PROBLEMS

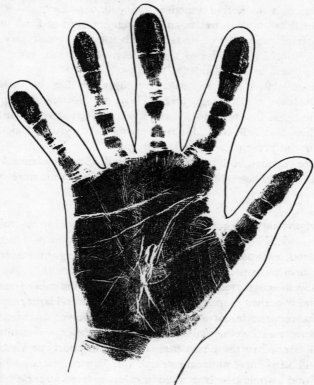

Fig. 123

Problems of the urinary system include kidney and bladder disorders. Markings suggesting a tendency to ailments in connection with the urinary system include:

1. A Luna mount cross-hatched with fine lines.

2. A vertical line running down the percussion side of the Mercury mount.
3. A yellowish scarring or small callus-like cluster of hard skin close to the outer side of the Life line as illustrated.

- Infection of the kidneys can cause serious long-term damage. If infection is suspected a doctor should be consulted immediately.
- Amongst the herbal remedies available, dandelion and stinging nettle are both diuretics and as such are used to flush out the system; rupture-wort eases inflammation of the urinary tract; traditionally, bladderwort has been used as a remedy for disorders of the bladder.
- A collection of tissue salts are suggested for the variety of disorders in this category. Ferr. Phos., Nat. Mur. and Mag. Phos. for stress incontinence; these three again, together with Kali. Phos. and Kali. Mur., for the treatment of cystitis; Calc. Phos. for the prevention of bed-wetting.
- Live yoghurt, both eaten as well as applied to the external areas, will help relieve and cool the irritation that accompanies cystitis.

VITALITY
Energy, vitality and a healthy constitution is marked in several ways:

1. Good, well-padded and springy mounts giving the whole hand a firm but resilient feel to it.
2. A well-constructed and well-endowed base to the palm. The thenar and hypothenar areas (the mounts of Venus and Luna) represent the repositories of energy and physical power, so when well-developed the two mounts together denote plenty of stamina and vigour. When these two appear weak and poorly padded, there will be a lack of physical strength and poor recuperative powers.
3. Good, strong, clearly marked lines in the hand, especially so the line of Life.
4. An indication of physical vitality and healthy resistance to disease may be seen on the back of the hand when the thumb is pressed against the palm. Vitality, resistance and recuperative powers are good if the muscle at the base of the 'v' that forms the join between thumb and palm is firm and springy when it humps up as the thumb is pressed against the edge of the palm.

When this muscle is flaccid or, instead of a hump, produces a depression, the general state of the constitution may be considered at a low ebb.

- Ginseng is held to boost strength and vitality. There are many herbal teas and preparations which have a stimulant action. Amongst these tonics are schisandra, pollen, sage and ginger.

VITAMIN AND MINERAL DEFICIENCIES

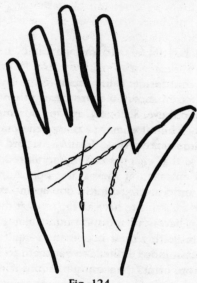

Fig. 124

1. Broken ridge patterns suggest vitamin deficiency.
2. Chains in the Life, Head and Heart lines may denote a mineral imbalance.
3. White specks on the nails can denote calcium or zinc imbalances.
4. Distortions, irregular growth, vertical or horizontal ridging, or nails that are either concave or convex in shape, all point to nutritional deficiencies and mineral imbalances.

See also **Nutritional Deficiencies**

APPENDIX

TAKING HANDPRINTS

Taking regular handprints is important for several reasons. Firstly, fine markings often show up more clearly than might be picked up with the naked eye. Secondly, any measurements are easier to take, especially when it comes to timing the major lines. Thirdly, and most importantly, they form a record of growth and development so that changes can be monitored and, if necessary, preventive action taken at the earliest opportunity.

The actual process of taking a handprint is a rather messy business so it's advisable to have all the tools at the ready. Children, of course, love having their handprints taken and there's usually no difficulty in getting their cooperation – quite the contrary, in fact, as it is often more difficult to get them to stop and you end up with far more prints than you need! And if you're taking your own handprints it's odds on that the phone will ring just when you're nicely inked up!

Using water-soluble lino-printing inks makes the whole thing a lot easier and means that you won't have to use solvents as the ink simply washes off with soap and water. So, if you could fill a basin with warm water before you begin, so much the better. The lino-printing ink that is recommended is fairly thick and comes in a tube. Some people make the mistake of using the more liquid printer's ink, or even fountain-pen ink that comes in a glass bottle. Neither are satisfactory for this purpose and are not recommended. Ink-pads are useful for taking individual fingerprints but again this ink will require a solvent to remove it.

Though lino-printing ink is fairly easy to come by in art shops, if you really can't get hold of a tube there are several household products that would substitute. Lipstick or waxy shoe-polish can give very satisfactory results, as long as they are not applied too thickly. Removing them from the hand, though, can be a problem.

EQUIPMENT

Recommended	Substitutes
• Lino printing ink	Lipstick, waxy shoe-polish
• Printer's roller	Rolling pin, empty bottle
• A sheet of glass	Formica board, piece of kitchen foil
• A4 paper	—
• Table knife	—
• Sharp pencil	—
• Square of foam rubber	Folded towel
• Tissues/cotton-wool	—

1. Squeeze a small amount of ink onto the glass/formica/foil and roll out thinly with the roller, or the empty bottle/rolling pin wrapped in clingfilm.
2. Roll the inked roller evenly all over the fingers, palm, and down to cover about the first 2–3 cm of the wrist. If using lipstick or shoe-polish apply thinly with tissues or cotton-wool.
3. Place the sheet of paper over the foam/folded towel and place the hand in as natural or comfortable a position as possible on the paper. If, on lifting up the hand, the central part of the palm has not printed, try the following alternatives. Remove the foam and place the paper directly on the table. Re-ink the hand and place it on the paper, then slip the table knife underneath the paper and press up into the hollow of the palm. If that doesn't work, a last resort that should get results is to work the other way up: when the hand has been re-inked, place it on the table palm-side up and carefully lay the paper on top, firmly pressing it into the hand. With this method you must ensure that you don't move the paper as you press it into the palm or else the print will smudge.
4. Whichever method is used, several clear prints of each hand should be taken. Each palmprint should be carefully marked

with the date, the owner's name, date of birth, sex and whether right- or left-handed.

5. When the hands are washed and dried and the inked print is also dry, re-position the hand over each print and draw around the outline with a sharp pen or biro. The advantage of taking the print on the hard table top without a sponge or towel underneath is that the outline can be pencilled in then and there.

PHOTOCOPIES

Modern photocopying machines can give excellent results if used as a back-up to inked handprints. However, as a sole source for analysis, a photocopy of a hand will not give enough of the fine detail that is required. In addition, the shape can easily be distorted if the hand is rested too heavily on the glass.

INDEX

diabetes 35, 37, 39
diet 16, 18, 29, 44, 51, 89, 97, 117, 135,
  170, 175, 193, 202, 203, 216, 217,
  222, 224, 228, 236
dietary deficiency 48, 69
digestive process 27, 28, 59, 166, 167,
  202, 210-11, 233
Down's Syndrome 33, 67-8, 129, 213
dyspepsia 167, 174, 221

Earth hand 4-6, 81, 82-3, 88, 124, 161
emphysema 5
empty hand 76-8
endocrine system 1, 40, 177-80, 200,
  235
endorphins 123
eyes 200, 211-12

familial tremor 37
Fate line 98, 99, 101-3, 104, 121, 135,
  138, 150-62
fatigue 5, 8, 165, 187, 189
Ferr. Phos. (Phosphate of Iron) ix, 205,
  206, 208, 212, 213, 215, 227, 236
ferrous sulphate 236
feverish condition 10, 26, 27, 28, 31, 39,
  41, 52, 89, 132, 137, 212-13
fingerprints 1, 3, 33, 56, 140
Fire hand 4, 9-11, 81, 85-6, 124, 161
Folic acid 89
free will 75
full hand 76-80, 209, 221

gall-bladder 167, 200, 211, 219, 233
gastric 174
genetics 1, 33, 65, 68, 108, 123, 129,
  132, 141, 145, 199, 216, 217
German measles 65
Girdle of Venus 103, 105, 168-70
glandular disorders 38
gout 39, 53, 227
gynaecological problems 24, 115, 165,
  168, 213-14

haemorrhoids 30
Head line 71, 80, 93, 95, 97, 99, 100-1,
  102, 103, 104, 107-8, 115, 121,
  122-39, 145, 146, 150, 151, 168, 171,
  180, 200, 209, 211, 214, 215, 217, 220,
  221, 225, 226, 231, 232, 239
headaches 8, 9, 14, 132, 137, 163-8,
  187, 215, 231

Health line 214, 219
hearing problems 146, 214-15
heart attack 51
heart disease 26, 31, 50, 54, 61, 69, 140,
  145, 227
Heart line 11, 71, 93, 97, 99, 103, 104,
  108, 109, 121, 138, 139-50, 151, 159,
  165, 169, 171, 200, 207, 208, 211, 215,
  217, 225, 228, 229, 239
Hepatica/liver line 103, 105 (*see also*
  Health line)
hepatitis 40
hernia 180, 218, 233
herpes simplex 219
high blood pressure 14, 38, 55, 56, 216,
  217, 218 (*see also* hypertension)
Hippocrates 33, 41, 43, 50
Hippocratic nail 50-1
HIV 203
hormones 123, 137, 177-80, 209, 234
hyperactivity 132, 170, 234
hypertension 17, 29, 41, 59, 179, 192-3,
  232 (*see also* high blood pressure)
hyperthyroidism 36 (*see also* thyroid)
hypochondira 46, 169
hypoglycaemia 37
hypothyroidism 53 (*see also* thyroid)
hysterectomy 180, 233

immune system 18, 167, 203
impotence 113
index finger 20, 28, 139, 143, 176, 178
indigestion 165, 189
injuries 10
insanity 24
insomnia 6, 147, 229-30
intestinal problems 5, 14, 24, 26, 27, 28,
  29, 32, 59, 148, 165, 174, 202, 210,
  211
iron 236
iron deficiency 89
island 29, 93, 97, 110, 115, 114-15, 124,
  133-5, 145-6, 160, 166-7, 171-2, 180,
  205, 207, 209, 211, 215, 226, 231

jaundice 40, 55, 89
joints 5

Kali. Mur. (Potassium Chloride) ix, 211,
  214, 215, 227, 238
Kali. Phos. (Potassium Phosphate) ix, 206,
  210, 212, 214, 215, 218, 222, 230, 231,
  236, 238